THE ANTI-CANCER
FOOD AND
SUPPLEMENT GUIDE

THE ANTI-CANCER FOOD AND SUPPLEMENT GUIDE

Debora Yost

A Lynn Sonberg Book

St. Martin's Paperbacks

Notice: This book is intended as a reference volume only, not as a medical manual. The information given here is designed to help you make informed decisions about your health. It is not intended as a substitute for any treatment that may have been prescribed by your doctor. If you suspect that you have a medical problem, we urge you to seek competent medical help.

Mention of specific companies, organizations, or authorities in the book does not imply endorsement by the author or publisher, nor does mention of specific companies, organizations, or authorities imply that they endorse this book, its author, or the publisher.

Internet addresses given in this book were accurate at the time it went to press.

THE ANTI-CANCER FOOD AND SUPPLEMENT GUIDE

Copyright © 2010 by Lynn Sonberg Book Associates.

Cover photo of carrots by Imagesource/Getty Images.

All rights reserved.

For information address St. Martin's Press, 175 Fifth Avenue, New York, NY 10010.

EAN: 978-0-312-37318-4

Printed in the United States of America

St. Martin's Paperbacks edition / April 2010

St. Martin's Paperbacks are published by St. Martin's Press, 175 Fifth Avenue, New York, NY 10010.

10 9 8 7 6 5 4 3 2 1

CONTENTS

CHAPTER 1

Preventing Cancer Today

"Genes are absolutely not our fate."

J. Craig Venter, Ph.D.

There is much we can do to prevent cancer.

If you find this hard to believe, consider this: Only 5 to 10 percent of all cancer cases can be attributed to genetics, says Craig Venter, Ph.D., one of the world's most prominent genetic scientists, and other leading cancer researchers from around the world. The other 90 to 95 percent have their roots in the environment and are largely under our control. In other words, we can radically lower our cancer risk by choosing to change the way we live our lives.

Nevertheless, cancer continues to be a worldwide killer. According to recent statistics, cancer accounts for approximately 23 percent of all deaths in the United States and is the second leading cause of death next to heart disease. And while death rates from cancer have been gradually declining during the last 30 years—thanks to prevention, early detection and better treatment—the worldwide incidence continues to grow. And the greatest increase is taking place in developing nations.

Ask scientists why this is happening and they will point West. As developing nations adopt a Western style of living, they are also adopting Western-style cancers, including lung, colorectal, breast, and prostate cancers. Our chances of getting cancer are not determined by the country from which we come, but by the way in which we choose to live. "Most of the world's cancer burden can be attributable to a few preventable risk factors," reports the International Agency for Research on Cancer (IARC) in its book, *World Cancer Report 2008*. And a preponderance of them involves our diet, lifestyle and what's happening in our environment.

Scientists maintain—and have plenty of evidence to prove it—that 90 percent of the world's cancer is caused by three environmental factors:

- Use of tobacco
- Poor dietary choices
- Sedentary and other lifestyle habits

If the world stopped smoking, say scientists, 30 percent of the world's cancer would go away. If we changed the way we eat—if we would eat more fruits and vegetables and less cured food and red meat—we could start to diminish another 30 percent of the world's cancer problem. We could help fight another 30 percent by getting more exercise, losing weight, drinking less, reducing pollution, and avoiding the sun and other sources of radiation.

This book is your roadmap to help you cancer-proof your life.

The main goal of a cancer prevention program is

to avoid the harmful elements in your environment that could eventually lead to cancer 20 or so years down the road. We know a great deal about risk factors for various kinds of cancer, based on research studies conducted over the last few decades, and chapter 2 presents the highlights, so that you will be able to identify your own risk factors.

Cancer is not one but a group of diseases in which mutant cells get damaged, grow out of control, and clump together as tumors. Normal, healthy cells don't do this. When they get damaged, they self-destruct and replicate into new, healthy cells. Carcinogens are continually challenging our healthy cells. Most of the time our immune system can fight them off. In some cases, carcinogens defeat immune-protecting resistance and cause cells to act abnormally. It takes years and often decades, however, for these cells to show themselves as cancer. This is why early detection programs are so important.

In the last decade or so, medical science has made remarkable strides in cancer screening techniques. Screening programs exist for many types of cancer, including three of the four major threats—breast, colorectal and prostate cancers. Chapter 3 introduces these programs and gives you the vital information you need to get your screenings on time.

Food is one of the most powerful weapons we have to fortify our immune systems against carcinogens. Scientists have identified 25,000 different phytochemicals in natural plant foods, mostly fruits and vegetables, with the potential to fight certain types of cancers. These phytochemicals are important to a cancer prevention program because they have the ability to track and help kill cancer cells. Studies show some of these nutrients are so powerful that they can help diminish the progression of advanced tumors and may even prevent them from migrating to other organs. Chapter 4 profiles nutrient-rich foods that have been scientifically shown to be cancer-fighting superstars.

Scientific studies have also found that some of the nutrients in these foods work just as well or even better when taken as supplements. Chapter 5 is your guide to the cancer-fighting supplements that are at the forefront of research.

Cancer prevention is not just about eating better, or taking a supplement, or making one or two little changes in your life. Preventing cancer is a *lifestyle*. This is what Chapter 6 is all about. It offers advice on how to change your life for the better, from getting more physically active to getting more environmentally active, including stomping out the biggest threat of all—tobacco.

What we eat, how we fortify our immune systems, and the lifestyles we choose form the strongest defensive system that any one person can undertake. If we all get in it together, we could prove the scientists are right and agree: Cancer *is* 90 percent preventable.

CHAPTER 2

What's Your Risk?

Right now, your best chance of conquering cancer is by preventing it. This means recognizing the known risk factors, determining your own personal risks, then taking the necessary action to reduce them.

The following questions address the major risk factors that, at least in some way, are in your control. Review them in the context of your own lifestyle. Being aware of your risk factors, and taking the necessary steps or precautions to reduce them, is key to your anti-cancer program.

1. DO YOU USE TOBACCO?

If you have any doubts that tobacco causes cancer, consider this: At the beginning of the twentieth century, before smoking came into vogue, lung cancer was extremely rare. Today, it is the biggest cause of cancer deaths throughout the world, and tobacco is accountable for 80 percent of them.

In fact, tobacco—whether you smoke it or chew it—is considered the number one preventable cause of premature death throughout the world. Experts estimate that if everyone quit smoking, the overall death rate from cancer would plummet 30 percent.

Americans are not the biggest smokers in the world, but we pay the heaviest price. Lung cancer is the number one cancer killer of both men and women in the United States, and U.S. women have the dubious distinction of having the second highest incidence of the disease in the world.

Tobacco, however, does not just put you at risk for lung cancer. Of the 4,800 particulate compounds that exist in smoking tobacco, 66 of them are proven carcinogens that have been linked to 13 different types of cancer. For example, smoking is the number one known cause of bladder cancer and is believed to be responsible for approximately 60 percent of all cases. Smoking is directly responsible for 20 percent of kidney cancer in men and 10 percent in women. A smoker's risk of kidney cancer is 50 percent greater than someone who never smoked and there is overwhelming evidence that tobacco is responsible for 30 percent of pancreatic cancer. So, enough. You're getting the point!

Smoking is linked to these cancers:

- Bladder
- Cervical
- Esophageal
- Kidney
- Laryngeal
- Liver
- Lung
- Myeloid leukemia
- Nasal
- Oral cavity
- Pancreatic

- Pharyngeal
- Stomach

WHY "LIGHT" CIGARETTES AREN'T WORKING

Cigarette manufacturers hoped to curb the cancer-causing effects of smoking by reducing the number of nitrosamines, the substances among the 66 known carcinogens in tobacco that cause the most danger.

So-called "light" cigarettes did cause people to modify their smoking, but not in a positive way. They actually encourage people to inhale deeper in order to feel the effect. Inhaling deeper means carcinogens reach deeper into the bronchial tubes.

Light cigarettes seem to have caused an unintentional backlash, as well. "U.S. blends of tobacco used to make cigarettes in more recent years may have increased the formation of nitrosamines during tobacco storage, processing and smoking," reports the IARC in its most recent *World Cancer Report.*

TAKE ACTION
If you smoke, your risk of getting cancer rises in proportion to the length of time you've been smoking, the number of cigarettes you smoke per day, and how deeply you inhale. Of the three, however, the number of years you've been smoking increases your risk the most. And it doesn't matter what you smoke. Smoking cigars or a pipe, whether you inhale or not, is just as harmful as cigarettes.

Now for the good news: *It's never too late to stop smoking.* Your cancer risk starts to decline the moment you put out your last cigarette. And if you quit smoking before middle age, you will avoid much of the lifetime risk you will incur if you continue to smoke. Relative risk markedly declines after five years and gradually continues to go down thereafter.

Smoking is a tough addiction to conquer, but successfully beating it offers totally positive benefits. There are plenty of smoking cessation programs aimed at helping smokers quit. Some work better than others. Chapter 6 reviews the programs that have been found to have the best odds for success. And in chapter 4, you'll find that there are certain foods that help neutralize the carcinogenic effects of tobacco.

2. DO YOU LIVE, WORK, OR SOCIALIZE WITH PEOPLE WHO SMOKE?

Nearly half of the people in the United States who don't smoke are exposed to people who do, which unnecessarily puts them at risk for any variety of respiratory illnesses, including lung caner. According to the American Cancer Society (ACS), secondhand smoke kills approximately 53,000 nonsmokers a year and 10 to 15 percent of lung cancers in people who never smoked are attributed to secondhand, or passive, smoking. This deleterious consequence is the result of nonsmokers involuntarily breathing in exhaled cigarette or cigar smoke.

Researchers found proof positive that one person's cigarette puts another's life in danger when they found they could detect cotinine, a byproduct of nicotine, in the blood and urine of nonsmokers exposed to tobacco smoke. They found further proof when they showed that blood levels of cotinine in nonsmokers have come down markedly in countries where there is a nationwide ban on smoking in public places. Studies of nonsmokers with lung cancer show that the most common exposure to secondhand smoke comes from three main sources: spouse, workplace, and social settings.

Several studies published since 2002 have linked secondhand smoke to these cancers:

- Cervical
- Childhood leukemia
- Kidney
- Lung
- Pancreatic
- Upper digestive tract
- Urinary-bladder

TAKE ACTION

If you live with someone who smokes or in a community with limited or no anti-smoking regulations, you are at increased risk for the side effects of secondhand smoke. This includes a lot of people because only an estimated 50 percent of Americans are shielded from noxious smoke in some way, such as through partial bans in restaurants and workplaces, or more widespread bans that include all public places. Bans in the United States are enforced on the local and state levels.

Your best defense against secondhand smoke is to get proactive about smoking bans in public (and, if needed, in your home). Chapter 6 offers important information about the positive effects of smoking bans around the world and the effects that can be achieved closer to home.

3. ARE YOU OVERWEIGHT OR OBESE?

Next to smoking, obesity is the largest cause of disease and premature death and it is escalating so rapidly that it is considered epidemic, not just in the United States, but around the world. This is significant because overweight and obesity are implicated in 40 percent of all cancers.

When it comes to cancer risk, overweight appears to be of significantly greater concern to women. Studies consistently show that overweight after menopause increases the risk of breast cancer and is highest in overweight women who have taken hormone replacement therapy. Overweight is also associated with an increased risk in ovarian cancer and endometrial cancer. In all, overweight and obesity are associated with an increased risk of these cancers:

- Breast (after menopause)
- Colorectal (men only)
- Endometrial
- Esophageal
- Gallbladder
- Kidney
- Leukemia
- Non-Hodgkins lymphoma
- Ovarian
- Pancreatic
- Prostate

TAKE ACTION

If you are overweight, following the recommendations in this book—most notably eating the foods and following the guidelines in chapter 4—should help you shed excess pounds naturally. Chapter 6 offers other helpful advice on how to lose and control excess weight. You'll even learn how to assess your cancer risk as it relates to your weight based on the same parameters used by scientists.

4. DO YOU LIVE AND WORK A SEDENTARY LIFESTYLE?

Numerous studies show a relationship between physical activity and cancer risk. There is evidence that cancer risk drops as amount of physical activity increases. There is also evidence linking a sedentary lifestyle as a separate risk factor for certain cancers. In fact, one study found that the risk of endometrial cancer rises with the number of hours a woman sits inactive during the course of a day.

Lack of exercise is most strongly linked to an increase in two major cancers, breast and colorectal. If you don't exercise at least moderately a minimum of three to five times a week, you are at greater risk for these cancers:

- Breast
- Colorectal cancer
- Endometrial
- Prostate

TAKE ACTION

It goes without saying that if you don't get any exercise, you need to start. This is especially true if you have a job that requires you to sit behind a desk most of the day. Chapter 6 offers more specific information on exercise and cancer risk and tells you exactly what you need to do to help reduce that risk.

5. DO YOU EAT LESS THAN FOUR OR FIVE SERVINGS OF FRUITS AND VEGETABLES A DAY?

Studies consistently find that as consumption of fruits and vegetables goes up, cancer risk comes down. This is particularly true for colorectal cancer, which is most strongly linked to diet.

Studies have found that a diet consistently *lacking* in fruits and vegetables is linked to these cancers:

- Cervical
- Esophageal
- Kidney
- Oral cavity
- Pharyngeal

TAKE ACTION

The ACS recommends that you get a minimum of four or five servings of fruits and vegetables a day as an overall hedge against all forms of cancer. While it does not specifically recommend what these fruits and vegetables should be, studies have identified at least 40 different foods containing anti-cancer nutritients. You'll find these foods, along with some great ideas on how to enjoy them, in chapter 4.

6. DO YOU BINGE DRINK OR DRINK EXCESSIVELY?

When it comes to health risk, drinking is a conundrum. The protective benefits of moderate drinking against heart disease are well known, but the pros and cons of drinking are muddled where cancer is concerned.

For example, moderate drinking—that means, two

drinks a day for men and one for women—has been found to be protective against ovarian and kidney cancers and non-Hodgkins lymphoma, but excessive drinking has been linked to an increased risk for nine types of cancer, including stomach and pancreatic cancers. And *any* drinking has been linked to an increased risk of breast and possibly colorectal cancers. In fact, 50 percent of all alcohol-related cancers in women are breast cancer. Some statistics show that each daily drink accounts for about a 7 percent higher breast cancer risk.

Here is the fact most important to consider in terms of your own drinking habits: Studies show that relative risk for cancer rises with the amount of alcohol you consume up to the equivalent of about a liter of wine or 8 ounces of hard liquor a day. You don't have to be a daily drinker, however, to be at risk for cancer. In fact, binge drinkers are considered to be at the highest risk of all, especially for pancreatic cancer.

Drinking increases the risks for these cancers:

- Breast
- Colorectal
- Esophageal
- Laryngeal
- Liver
- Oral cavity
- Non-malignant skin cancer
- Pancreatic
- Pharyngeal
- Stomach

TAKE ACTION

When it comes to alcohol and cancer, what you drink and how much you drink matters—a lot. Chapter 6 offers details on how best to fit alcohol into an anti-cancer lifestyle, including the types of alcohol to avoid and who should avoid it. You'll find more information on drinking habits and their relationship to cancer in chapters 4 and 6.

7. DO YOU SMOKE AND DRINK?

Smoking and drinking independently have their own way of increasing your cancer risk, but together they are double trouble. Though smoking is the greater risk of the two, research in the early 1970s found that the two together increase cancer risk more than either one alone. Although the exact mechanism is not known, researchers believe drinking somehow works synergistically to augment the carcinogenic effects of tobacco. Smoking and drinking, in fact, account for 90 percent of all cancers of the larynx. Smoking also aggravates the effects of alcohol on the liver.

Habitual smoking and drinking are linked to an increased risk for these cancers:

- Bladder
- Cervical
- Kidney
- Liver
- Lung
- Nasal
- Oral cavity
- Pancreatic
- Stomach
- Myeloid leukemia

TAKE ACTION
Obviously, smoking and drinking don't mix. If you drink, you should not smoke, and you should stay away from people who do.

8. DID YOU EXPERIENCE SUNBURN AS A CHILD?
Radiation from the sun is the main cause of skin cancer and your risk of getting it is programmed in your genes—the ones that determine your skin's ability to burn or tan. Though no one is immune to the damaging effects of the sun, those most susceptible to all types of skin cancer are fair-skinned, freckled, red-haired individuals who burn easily—and got sunburned as a child. This profile is the cause of 80 percent of melanomas, the worst and most deadly form of skin cancer. In fact, if you never experienced reddening from exposure to the sun in your first 15 to 20 years of life, your risk of getting melanoma during adulthood is almost zero.

People with darker skin, such as Hispanics, Indians, and those of Italian decent, are not at as great a risk, and skin cancer is rare, though not unheard of, in African Americans. Their burn protection comes from a pigment in the skin called melanin, which is synthesized by exposure to the ultraviolet radiation from the sun. The more melanin that is manufactured, the darker the skin gets. Caucasians call it a tan; doctors call it sun-damaged skin.

Non-melanoma skin cancer by far is seen more than melanoma. It comes in two forms: squamous cell carcinoma, which occurs almost exclusively on chronically exposed areas of the skin and is caused by cumulative sun exposure, and basal cell carcinoma, which can show up on parts of the body that have rarely seen the sun.

Next to the fairness of your skin, your geographic

location is your next measure of risk. Climate, altitude, latitude, and distance from the equator all factor into the equation. Skin cancer is most common where the sun is brightest. It affects 50 percent of the population in tropical Queensland, Australia, which has the highest incidence of skin cancer in the world. The alpine regions of Switzerland also have a high rate of skin cancer. Southeast Arizona is the skin cancer capital of the United States.

TANNING BEDS ARE MORE DANGEROUS THAN THE SUN

For many years scientists believed that all the sun's harmful effects come from the UVB rays that filter through the sun's protective ozone layer. These are the rays that cause the burn and make the tan. More recently, however, scientists found that UVA rays are also carcinogenic. Even though it takes a lot more UVA rays to cause harm, the damage penetrates deeper into the skin.

This is what makes tanning beds so potentially deadly. Some tanning units can produce ultraviolet ray intensity 10 to 15 times greater than the noonday sun on a sunny summer day in Australia and UVA doses can be as much as four times that of the natural sun.

"Such powerful sources of UVA radiation probably do not exist on the Earth's surface, and repeated exposures to high doses of UVA constitute a new phenomenon in humans," says the IARC.

Studies have found that women younger than 30 who expose their skin to the unnatural rays of tanning beds increase their risk of melanoma later in life by 70 percent.

TAKE ACTION

Your risk of getting skin cancer is largely determined by how you live with the sun. There are two types of so-called sun behaviors. Non-intentional sun exposure describes the person who walks, works, exercises or hobbies in the sun wearing typical attire. How you dress, where you live, and your compliance in using sunscreen determines how often certain parts of the skin get unprotected, cumulative exposure to harmful rays. This makes you more vulnerable to basal cell and squamous cell skin cancers.

Intentional exposure describes people who bask in the sun in bathing suits for the express purpose of getting a tan. Experts say that sporadic, intense exposure to the sun—a once-a-year weekly beach vacation, for example—puts you at high risk. These are the people most vulnerable to all forms of skin cancer, including melanoma.

Chapter 6 offers detailed advice on how to protect your skin type from a harmful burn and what you should do to reduce your risk of skin cancer. While there are precautions you can take to protect yourself from the harmful ultraviolet rays of the sun, there is only one precaution necessary when it comes to tanning beds and tanning salons: Avoid them!

9. HAVE YOU HAD EXCESSIVE EXPOSURE TO X-RAYS OR OTHER FORMS OF IONIZING RADIATION?

Ionizing radiation—that is, radiation powerful enough to break chemical bonds—is the most studied and scrutinized of all known carcinogens. It is impossible to avoid and we all carry minute amounts in our bodies.

We get doses from the sun. We get it from radioactivity in rocks and soil, and from radon that seeps into our

homes and office buildings. We get it from weapons
testing fallout and routine releases from nuclear instal-
lations that get into the atmosphere. Virtually everyone
is exposed to it sometime during their medical life as a
result of diagnostic X-rays, computerized tomography
(CT) scans and nuclear medicine.

Scientists assure us that the amount of ionizing radiation the typical American is exposed to is not enough
to accumulate into a lifetime risk of cancer. Recently,
however, concern has been raised over the amount of
radiation Americans are getting as a result of medical
imaging procedures. A major study conducted in 2006
found that Americans are being exposed to more than
seven times as much ionizing radiation from medical
procedures than they were during the early 1980s, an
amount that caused the National Council on Radiation
Protection and Measures to raise the caution flag. Ionizing radiation has been linked to these cancers:

- Bone
- Breast
- Leukemia
- Liver
- Lung
- Thyroid

TAKE ACTION
Though most Americans do not get enough exposure to
radiation to measure up to a lifetime risk, there are actions you can take to minimize your exposure. In chapter 6 you'll find guidelines on making wise choices
concerning X-rays and other medical procedures.

10. DO YOU KNOW IF YOU ARE GETTING RADON IN YOUR HOME?

Next to cigarettes, radon is the second leading cause of lung cancer and kills an estimated 20,000 Americans a year. The U.S. Environmental Protection Agency (EPA) considers it a national health problem.

Radon is an invisible, odorless natural radioactive gas. It results from the natural decay of uranium in soil, rock, and water. And it seeps into homes and buildings from the ground. It is measured in picocuries per liter (pCi/L). The EPA considers no levels safe, but Congress has established an acceptable level to be 4pCi/L—a level some experts say is equal to smoking a half pack of cigarettes a day. An estimated 8 million homes—one in five—in the United States have radon above this level. All states are affected, although New Jersey, Pennsylvania, and upstate New York are among the areas with the highest concentrations.

Uranium is also found in granite and the explosion in the popularity of granite countertops, walls, floors, and mantels in homes has raised concern about radon. Several studies have verified that granite countertops do emit radon, but most experts agree that the amount is minimal.

Radon is associated with this cancer:

• Lung

TAKE ACTION

Radon testing is easy and inexpensive—something you can do on your own. Chapter 6 offers details on how to test for radon and what to do about it if levels are too high.

11. DO YOU LIVE IN OR NEAR A BIG CITY OFTEN CAST IN SMOG?

It's been established for decades that long-term exposure to tiny particles of dust and soot in air from factories, cars, and power plants—in other words, air pollution—is a health risk, and the EPA has established reefs of regulations to keep it under control. As a result, the risk of cancer from breathing bad air is small.

Nevertheless, you can't escape pollution. Carcinogens and possible carcinogens are part of the environment, and we all carry traces of them in our bodies. There is great disparity, however, in the quality of air from one place to another. And the places where air quality is poorest—and risk is greatest—are urban areas containing coal-fired power plants, petroleum refineries, metal manufacturing plants, iron refineries, incinerators, and smelters. There is abundant evidence that lung cancer rates are higher in cities than in rural areas and highest in cities with the most pollution.

The greatest risk from what's in the air is any variety of respiratory illnesses, but cancer experts agree that risk rises with exposure to particular atmospheric pollutants, including benzopyrene, benzene, some metals, particulate matter, and ozone.

Our understanding of ozone's carcinogenic capacity was raised substantially in 2009 with the results of the first long-term nationwide study on the effects of ground-level ozone. The study, involving 450,000 people and spanning 18 years, found that those exposed to ground-level ozone had an average 30 percent greater risk of dying from lung disease, including lung cancer.

Ground-level ozone—in other words, smog—results when nitrogen dioxide from tailpipes, coal-fired power plants, and other industries collides with oxygen in the presence of sun. Prior to 2009 it was considered a secondary pollution because it takes time to form. The new study found unsafe levels of ground-level ozone in 96 American metropolitan areas, including many in compliance with the EPA's short-term ozone standards.

While air pollution is most prevalent at its source— the inner city, industrial areas, and along crowded roadways—ground level ozone tends to concentrate in suburbs and rural areas downwind from the inner city.

Pollution has been linked to these cancers:

• Lung
• Lymphoma
• Kidney
• Testicular

TAKE ACTION

Human exposure to air pollution is hard to estimate but you can consider yourself at greater risk if you live near specific sources of pollution where different gaseous and particulate components comingle in the air you breathe. There is little you can do about the air in your environment short of moving. However, you can help fortify your resistance to these pollutants by eating more foods listed in chaper 4 and taking some of the supplements recommended in chapter 5. Also, chapter 6 offers tips that will help you identify the pollution rate in your home county.

12. DO YOU EAT A LOT OF RED OR PROCESSED MEAT OR GRILLED FOODS?

Numerous studies have been conducted in an effort to find out the role red meat and processed foods play in cancer risk. Results have been mixed, although there is enough evidence to indict eating red meat as a possible risk factor for some types of cancer. The largest body of evidence links meat consumption with colorectal cancer and, to a lesser degree, breast cancer. One study found that eating more than three ounces of meat a day increases the risk of colon cancer by 25 percent. Processed meat pushed the risk to 67 percent. In most of these studies, red meat included beef, pork, lamb and processed meats, such as ham, salami, bacon and charcuterie. Preserved meat processing involves potential cancer-causing nitrates and nitrites.

The bigger indictment concerning meat, however, comes from two cooking styles—fried and grilled over charcoal or on a gas grill at high temperatures. Grilling and frying foods at temperatures above 352°F cause molecules in meats to break and produce toxic substances called polycyclic aromatic hydrocarbons (PAHs). This includes all animal foods, even fish. For reasons no one can explain, PAHs do not form on grilled fruits and vegetables.

Eating meats cooked well done to the point of charring creates substances called heterocyclic aromatic amines (HAAs). When consumed, PAHs and HAAs have the ability to induce DNA damage in cells, which some scientists believe can lead to cancer. Researchers from the University of Minnesota School of Public Health found that people who prefer meat cooked well done had a 70 percent higher risk of pancreatic cancer than people who ate meat rare or medium rare. Charred meat is also associated with breast, colon and stomach cancer. One study found that people who eat the most barbecued red meat had almost double the number of precancerous colon polyps than people who did not eat grilled food.

Eating red meat and grilled meat and fish have been linked with these cancers:

- Breast
- Colorectal
- Endometrial
- Ovarian
- Pancreatic
- Stomach

Take Action
You don't have to give up meat or the grill. Chapter 4 offers sensible guidelines on meat consumption and tips on how to make grilling safer.

13. ARE YOU SEXUALLY ACTIVE WITH MULTIPLE PARTNERS?
Chronic infection is believed to be the cause of 18 percent of all cancers worldwide, and the virus responsible for the majority of them in the United States is the sexually transmitted human papillomavirus (HPV).

HPV is considered a known carcinogen. It is the leading cause of cervical cancer and is associated with an increased risk of six others. Virtually all cases of cervical cancer, however, are caused by persistent infection from HPV, the most common sexually transmitted infection in young adults. Both men and women can get the infection. In the majority of cases, the immune system fights off the virus and it dies out on its own without causing any harm. Only a small percentage of viruses evolve into cancer.

A vaccine to prevent HPV infection became available in 2007, but it is currently only available for women. It is not effective if the virus has already been contracted, which is why doctors recommend that young women get vaccinated before sexual activity begins. Whether or not the vaccine offers a lifetime of protection is yet to be known for certain.

Women who have HPV and take birth control pills are at increased risk for getting cervical cancer. The risk drops, however, when the Pill is stopped. Certain types of sexual activity can increase risk. Risk also rises for people with multiple sex partners and those who use non-barrier birth control.

HPV increases the risk of these cancers:

- Anal
- Cervical
- Non-malignant melanoma
- Oral cavity
- Penile
- Vaginal
- Vulvar

TAKE ACTION
Although sexually active women are at highest risk, it is important for all women to get screened for cervical cancer. You'll find the guidelines for cervical cancer screening in chapter 3 beginning on page 38.

14. HAVE YOU HAD STOMACH PROBLEMS OR ULCERS ASSOCIATED WITH THE *H. PYLORI* VIRUS?
Some cancer specialists theorize that if *Helicobacter pylori* would go away, 40 to 70 percent of stomach cancer would be eliminated.

Long-term infection with *H. pylori*, a common bacterium that causes gastritis and most ulcers, is estimated to be the cause of 63 percent of stomach cancers world-wide, though rates are coming down. In Japan, which has the highest rate of stomach cancer in the world, researchers in one study found that *H. pylori* was present in every case of stomach cancer.

H. pylori is associated with an increased risk of these cancers:

- Cervical
- Gallbladder
- Non-malignant skin
- Stomach

TAKE ACTION
H. pylori can be eliminated with antibiotics. If you have chronic gastrointestinal problems you should see a doctor, who can test you for a possible ulcer and treat you accordingly.

15. DO YOU HAVE DIABETES OR DOES IT RUN IN YOUR FAMILY?
Diabetes is bad news. Not only does it require life-altering scrutiny and attention to your diet, but it is implicated in an increased risk for certain types of cancer.

Two major national population studies, one in Sweden and the other in Denmark, found a correlation between Type 2 diabetes (also known as adult-onset diabetes) and the incidence of kidney cancer. According to the study, diabetes increases risk by 40 percent in men and 70 percent in women.

Chronically high levels of insulin in overweight women are associated with an increased risk of endometrial cancer. And a diet rich in carbohydrates with a high glycemic index—that is, foods that significantly raise blood glucose levels—is associated with an increase in the risk of ovarian and colorectal cancers. This includes white and brown sugars, honey, refined grains, and potatoes.

Cancers associated with diabetes and insulin are:

- Colorectal
- Endometrial
- Kidney
- Ovarian
- Pancreatic

TAKE ACTION

If you are at risk for diabetes, make sure you get your blood glucose level checked at least once a year as part of your yearly physical. Also, discuss your risk with your doctor, who may decide to check your blood glucose level more frequently. Overweight and heart disease are associated with an increased risk of diabetes. Also, diabetes can run in families.

16. DO YOU HAVE HIGH BLOOD PRESSURE?

For years, researchers had a hunch that there is a relationship between high blood pressure and cancer, but Israeli researchers put this to rest in 2002 after investigating cancer deaths in more than 47,000 people over the course of 34 years. They found a direct link to only one type of cancer—kidney. Another study found that the risk exists even in people who are successfully controlling their blood pressure with medication. Women with high blood pressure are more at risk than men, with a 39 percent increased risk of developing kidney cancer compared to a 21 percent risk in men.

TAKE ACTION

In addition to the efforts you are probably already taking to keep your blood pressure under control, you can avoid smoking, as it is a major risk factor for kidney cancer. The most common symptom of kidney cancer is blood in the urine.

17. DOES CANCER RUN IN YOUR FAMILY?

Cancer does tend to run in families, but just because you have a relative or relatives who have had cancer does not necessarily mean that you'll get it. One of the biggest mysteries associated with cancer is why some people at high risk for cancer never get it, while people at a low risk do—and this includes those who are genetically predisposed.

Keep in mind, that just because one or both parents had cancer, it does not mean the same cancer will happen to you.

Even if you inherited a cancer gene, it still doesn't mean that your fate is sealed. The gene must first be expressed, and research shows that environmental factors play a big role in both making it happen and preventing it from happening. In most cases, chances are small that the necessary combination of events will occur to allow a normal cell to progress into a fully malignant tumor.

When it all shakes out, inheritance accounts for only anywhere from 5 to 10 percent of all cancers.

In general, inherited forms of cancer frequently occur

at an earlier age—before 40 or 50. Most environmental damage takes decades to become cancerous.

On the positive side, it is also possible for you to inherit a natural ability to suppress cancer. There are individual differences in the ability to detoxify or metabolize carcinogens that, in part, are dictated by your genes.

Currently, biomarkers exist for these cancers: breast and ovarian (BRCA-1 and BRCA-2) and colon and endometrial cancers (MLH-1 and MLH-2). This means that if you possess a BRCA gene, you are at higher risk for both cancers. Same with the MLH genes.

Other cancers that can run in the family, to some degree, include bladder, brain, eye, kidney, lung, leukemia, lymphoma, nasopharyngeal, pancreatic, skin, stomach, and thyroid.

TAKE ACTION

If cancer tends to run in your family, practicing an anti-cancer lifestyle can help reduce the odds that you, too, may someday get the same cancer. Make it a point to keep a family record of illnesses and causes of death among your direct ancestors so it can be passed along to your own children and grandchildren. If there is cancer in your family, it is all the more important for you to get appropriately screened and to recognize symptoms. You'll find important information on screening, detection and genetic testing in chapter 3.

For example, if you come from a family in which one or more smokers died of lung cancer, it means you may have a higher risk of lung cancer *if* you are a smoker yourself. Likewise, skin cancer tends to run in families, especially those with a heritage of fair skin and red hair. If skin cancer runs in your family, it means it is important for you to take precautions in the sun.

Knowledge is awareness, which in and of itself is a form of prevention because it, hopefully, is incentive to follow an anti-cancer lifestyle. And that's what the rest of this book is all about.

CHAPTER 3

What You Should Know about Screening and Detection

Cancer is a stealthy intruder. It isn't something that develops suddenly, but it can seem that way when mysterious symptoms lead to a diagnosis of cancer. Some cancers give hints of their presence early on, while others present no symptoms until they have progressed to a potentially life-threatening stage.

There is no way to know your chance of getting cancer in your lifetime, but your best chance of beating the odds is by finding cancer as early as possible. Early detection and better treatment get most of the credit for the steady decline in cancer deaths over the last 30 years. And the biggest drop—26 percent—is among younger Americans. This is why screening is so important. It is an essential aspect of your medical care that will help you maintain quality of life for decades to come.

Every year, screening helps prevent millions of people from premature death due to cancer. The American Cancer Society (ACS) recommends screenings for only a handful of cancers but they include three out of the top four major killers—breast, colorectal and prostate cancers. For other common cancers, routine checkups, diligent attention to changes in the body, and speed in getting suspicious symptoms evaluated can also mean detecting cancer at an early stage. It is unequivocally established that survival is much greater for early, localized cancers than for late-stage, advanced forms of the disease.

Here is essential information about screening, detection, and diagnosis for nine of the more common cancers that strike Americans.

THE STAGES OF CANCER

Cancer prognosis and treatment is based on the stage of cancer at diagnosis, which ranges from early Stage 0 or Stage 1 to advanced Stage 4. How these stages are defined, however, can vary for particular cancers or type of cancer.

Stage systems are continually evolving as scientists learn more about different cancers. There are, however, common elements in classifying a cancer's stage. They are:

- Location of the primary tumor—that is, the organ where the cancer originally started, should it have already spread
- Tumor size and number of tumors
- Tumor type
- Lymph node involvement
- Presence or absence of metastasis—that is, if cancer has spread to other organs

So, if you or a loved one is diagnosed with cancer, ask the oncologist to explain in detail *all* the stages for this particular cancer and its treatment options.

BREAST CANCER SCREENING
The American Cancer Society recommends:

• *Yearly mammogram starting at age 40*
• *A breast exam as part of a medical exam every three years during a woman's 20s and 30s and every year for women 40 and older*

Mammograms save lives. This simple, relatively painless procedure can detect a tumor in the breast long before it can be felt or produce symptoms.

Breast cancer kills more women worldwide that any other form of cancer and is second only to lung cancer as the leading cause of cancer death among American women.

Getting a routine mammogram, however, can help bring this rate down. For 20 years, the ACS has been advising women to have a mammogram every year starting at age 40. Studies spanning 25 years and multiple countries have found that mammography screening reduced deaths from breast cancer among women ages 40 to 69 by 40 to 46 percent.

Despite these statistics, the U.S. government stirred controversy in late 2009 when it recommended screenings begin at age 50 and be repeated every other year until age 74, after which screening should be discontinued. At the time, the ACS and most doctors disagreed with the recommendations made by the U.S. Preventive Services Task Force, a panel of experts that advises doctors on medical procedures.

Nevertheless, only an estimated 62 percent of American women over age 40 are taking advantage of this life-saving screening.

Breast cancer is a disease in which malignant tumors form in the tissue of the breast. Though the exact cause of breast cancer is still unclear, numerous studies strongly suggest that there is a relationship between risk and high levels of the female hormone estrogen. Studies show that women with the highest levels of estrogen have about a two-thirds greater risk for breast cancer than women with the lowest levels.

Screening: What to Expect

Mammography is performed by a skilled technician using a special X-ray machine and film designed specifically to examine breast tissue. The only risk involved is exposure to ionizing radiation, but doctors consider it slight, especially compared to the benefit of catching life-threatening cancer at an early stage. Mammograms also create anxiety in many women that often doesn't go away until the results are in—one of the reasons the government used in recommending less-frequent testing.

During the procedure, which only takes about 20 minutes, the technician manually compresses each breast between two plates and takes pictures from a minimum of two angles—top to bottom and side to side. The film is then examined by a radiologist who looks for abnormal spots that could be a sign of a tumor. The results are sent to your doctor who should pass them on to you within a week or two.

Your first mammogram is considered your baseline and is used as a comparison for all future procedures. For this reason, it is important to use the same imaging center each year, if possible. If you move, you should get copies or have copies forwarded to the new radiological practice that you will be using. Being able to access your mammogram history is important to your care.

A mass can usually be detected through a mammogram before it can be felt. A tumor detected and treated at this stage offers the best possible opportunity for survival and is your best chance to have the tumor and the least amount of breast tissue removed during surgery.

Reading the results of a mammogram is subjective, but the risk that a radiologist will miss spotting a tumor is small—about 5 percent in the general population. Large-breasted women have the biggest chance of falling into that 5 percent risk.

Major Screening Risk: Fatty Breasts

Normal breast tissue appears white and opaque on an X-ray, but dense tissue appears dark and translucent. As a result, a tumor can be harder to spot. One of the few studies on mammography and dense tissue was conducted in Seattle over a five-year period among women with a family history of breast cancer. Follow-up found that radiologists missed detecting a tumor on X-rays 20 percent of the time in women with predominantly fatty breasts and 70 percent of the time in women with extremely fatty breast tissue.

More accurate readings can be found through a magnetic resonance imaging (MRI) scan, but this test is costly and not currently recommended except for women who meet these criteria:

- Women younger than 40 who have tested positive for carrying the BRCA-1 or BRCA-2 breast cancer gene.
- Women with a strong family history of breast or ovarian cancer and women who have been treated for Hodgkins disease.

A new high-tech screening method called molecular breast imaging (MBI) is currently being tested that will help identify a tumor in dense breast tissue that can be hard to detect through mammography. With MBI, a woman is given an injection of a short-lived radioactive substance that pools in tumor cells more than it does in normal cells. A radiologist can see so-called "hot spots" by means of a radiation-detecting camera.

In a 2009 study at Mayo Clinic, MBI detected three times as many cancers in women with dense breast tissue and an increased risk of breast cancer. Researchers also found that MBI produced fewer false positives, meaning results show an abnormality that turns out to be non-cancerous.

The problem with MBI is exposure to radiation. Before it can be introduced into general use, researchers need to reduce the dose of radiation currently required to perform the test.

Clinical Breast Exam

Even though mammograms are not recommended until age 40, the ACS says that breast cancer prevention should begin at the age of 20 with a yearly breast exam that is part of an annual physical or gynecological checkup. This is a painless manual exam in which the doctor feels and palpitates the breast, nipples and lymph nodes near and under the arm for lumps or bumps.

In addition, you also need to BSA—that is, Be Self Aware, meaning you should be familiar with how your breasts feel. At one time, the code was BSE, which stood for Breast Self Exam, which every woman was supposed to perform on herself in between doctor's visits. This, however, is no longer recommended. Leading cancer specialists found that many women were confused as to how to do the exam properly, so they didn't do it at all. Instead, doctors recommend that women become familiar with how their breasts feel. If anything looks or feels out of the ordinary, call your doctor right away for an appointment.

BSA of the Symptoms

Being self-aware also means knowing the symptoms that could indicate breast cancer. Realize, however, that symptoms of breast cancer can vary from woman to woman. Also, don't assume that finding a lump means you have cancer. Most lumps that are found are not cancer, but finding any of the following warrants an immediate call to your doctor.

- An odd-feeling mass or lump that did not exist before
- Enlargement of nodules in the armpit
- Changes in size, shape, texture, or color of the breast, such as redness or scaliness
- Changes in nipples, such as pulling to one side
- Discharge from nipple

Diagnosis and Treatment

Should a mammogram show a suspicious mass in breast tissue, your doctor may want to redo the mammogram or do another test, such as an MRI, but any suspicious lump is generally followed by a biopsy. A breast biopsy is a surgical procedure in which breast tissue is removed and examined by a pathologist.

Breast cancer is a complex disease and there are many factors involved in deciding the next course of action. For example, there are several different options for biopsy, which range from taking a small sample from the mass to removing the entire mass for examination. There are many treatment options as well, which should be dictated by the type of breast cancer and its stage of advancement.

There are four standard types of surgery:

1. Breast-sparing surgery (lumpectomy), in which just the tumor and a portion of healthy surrounding tissue are removed.
2. Partial mastectomy, in which the cancer and part of the breast surrounding the cancer are removed.
3. Total mastectomy, in which the entire cancerous breast is removed.
4. Modified radical mastectomy, which includes removal of lymph nodes under the arm, the lining over the chest muscles, and sometimes part of the chest wall muscles. Radiation therapy, chemotherapy, or hormone therapy may be warranted, depending on type of breast cancer and outcome of surgery.

High-Risk Profile

Many factors play into the risk for breast cancer, but a high-risk profile can be an older, overweight woman who does little exercise, eats a fatty diet and takes more than one alcoholic drink a day. She also may have had her first child after age 30, taken hormone replacement therapy for menopause (HRT) and had a mother, sister or daughter who had breast cancer.

One factor that appears to play into increased risk is a woman's cumulative number of lifetime ovulations. An example would be a childless woman who started menstruating before age 12, stopped after age 55, or had a menstrual cycle shorter or longer than the average 26–29 days. Ovulation is dependent on the production of estrogen, which is heavily implicated in the development of the disease.

Risk also goes up for women who have had previous female-related health conditions. A benign breast lump raises the risk slightly and having had ovarian cancer raises it significantly. The risk is two- to threefold higher for women who have had fibrocystic breast disease. Women with a family history of breast cancer who carry one of the two genetic mutations (BRCA-1 and BRCA-2) for the disease are at highest risk.

CERVICAL CANCER SCREENING
The American Cancer Society recommends:

- *A Pap test for cancer every year starting approximately three years after a woman begins having vaginal intercourse, but no later than age 21.*
- *A liquid-based test for presence of HPV infection every two years.*
- *At or after age 30, women who have had three normal test results in a row can reduce screening to every two or three years.*

Cervical cancer has dramatically declined in the United States over the last 60 years, thanks to a Greek doctor named Georgios Papanikolaou.

Dr. Papanikolaou invented a simple test that detects abnormal changes in the cervix, which over the course of 10 to 15 years can develop into cancer of the lining of the cervix. A Pap test can also detect changes in cervical cells, known as dysplasia, which over time can lead to cancer. Because of this test, called a Pap smear, this once deadly cancer is highly preventable. The primary cause of cervical cancer (95 percent) is persistent infection from the sexually transmitted human papillomavirus (HPV). The virus is so common that virtually every woman is exposed to it shortly after she starts sexual activity. In most cases, the virus disappears on its own, but for some unknown reason a small percentage of women are unable to fight off the infection. There are some 100 strains of HPV of which only about 15 stimulate growth of precancerous lesions. If infection persists without being detected and treated, these lesions gradually change into cancer. The cancer has been discovered in women as young as 30, although this is rare. Risk for the disease increases until about age 70. In fact, women 70 and older who have had three or more consecutive screenings in the last 10 years can stop cervical cancer screening. Screening after a total hysterectomy is not necessary unless the surgery was performed because of cervical cancer.

Screening: What to Expect

Most cervical abnormalities caused by HPV do not progress to the point of cancer, but for those that do, chances for successful treatment are highest when the disease is detected early. A Pap test is your insurance that it will be.

A Pap test is usually given as part of a woman's annual gynecological exam. It's a no-risk procedure that takes but a minute or two. During the procedure, a doctor or trained medical assistant inserts a tool called a speculum into the vagina and takes a collection of cells from the cervical lining. The cells are then sent to a lab for microscopic inspection and the results are reported back to your doctor, then to you, within a week or two. Reading the results of the test is subjective, and has an accuracy rate of 91 to 96 percent.

Diagnosis and Treatment

If a Pap test reveals suspicious lesions, your doctor will do a colposcopy, a diagnostic procedure that allows a close-up inspection of the area surrounding the abnormal tissue that cannot be seen by the naked eye. This is usually followed by a biopsy to remove sample tissue for microscopic examination. Biopsy for this cancer can be done in the doctor's office without anesthesia.

If the biopsy reveals advanced cancer, high-technology testing may be needed to see if the cancer has spread. This could include a chest X-ray, computed tomography (CT) scan, or magnetic resonance imaging (MRI).

Course of treatment depends on the stage of the cancer, size of the tumor and where a woman stands in her childbearing plans. It can range from laser-type surgery to remove precancerous or early-stage cancerous lesions to a hysterectomy to remove the uterus and cervix.

Radiation therapy can be used in place of surgery but is only recommended for women who have very large cancerous lesions or have cancer that has spread beyond the cervix. Chemotherapy is usually given along with radiation therapy.

What You Need to Know about HPV

The biggest advancement concerning cervical cancer since the Pap smear was the June 2006 introduction of a vaccine to prevent HPV infection. Scientists see it as a breakthrough that will dramatically reduce the risk of getting cervical cancer if females get the vaccine before starting sexual activity.

Because it is only effective before the onset of sexual activity, doctors recommend that mothers have their daughters vaccinated around the age of 11 or 12. The vaccine, which goes by the brand name Gardasil, currently is only available to females between the ages of 11 and 26, even though males are carriers of the virus, too. Because the vaccine is new, its long-term preventive effect is yet to be determined.

HPV does not only cause cervical cancer, but it can also cause cancers of the vagina, vulva, anus, penis, and oral cavity.

A Pap smear cannot confirm the presence of HPV, but there is another that can. This is called a liquid-based cytology test and is conducted in the same fashion and is done at the same time as a Pap test. The test is recommended every three years for women who:

- Started sexual activity before age 21
- Have or have had multiple sex partners
- Have been on oral contraceptives long term
- Have been infected with chlamydia, a common sexually transmitted disease

Recognize the Symptoms

There are no symptoms of the presence of HPV or the precancerous lesions that eventually turn into cancer. Symptoms do not appear until the cancer appears. If you experience one or more of these symptoms, call your doctor for an evaluation.

- Bleeding between periods
- Bleeding after sexual intercourse
- Recurrent urinary tract infections
- Vaginal discharge
- Heavy menstrual flows
- Backache
- Lower abdominal pain

HIGH-RISK PROFILE

A high-risk woman who started having sex as a teenager, has a history of multiple sexual partners, and uses non-barrier birth control methods, such as oral contraceptives. Smoking adds to the risk, as does having had a sexually transmitted disease.

COLORECTAL CANCER SCREENING

The American Cancer Society recommends:

• *Screening, preferably by colonoscopy, every 10 years starting at age 50. Less effective screenings should be done more frequently.*

It's a shame that one of the leading causes of cancer death is also one of the most preventable. An estimated 90 percent of colorectal cancer deaths could be prevented if everyone at the age of 50 would get the highly effective screening exam known as a colonoscopy. Yet, 40 percent of the people who should get a colonoscopy don't. Why? Mainly fear. But it is really fear of the unknown, because a colonoscopy is not as scary as some people think, says Dale Burleson, M.D., a colorectal surgeon at Baylor Medical Center in San Francisco.

Colorectal cancer occurs when cells in the colon or rectum grow uncontrollably and form lesions known as polyps. Most often these growths are small and noncancerous, but they can develop into cancer over time. A colonoscopy is the currently accepted standard and most widely used screening method for detecting precancerous and cancerous lesions in the small bowel and large colon. The procedure is considered the most effective way to prevent colorectal cancer and screen for symptoms.

Colonoscopy: What to Expect

A colonoscopy is a procedure in which a doctor inserts a long, flexible tube attached to a tiny camera into the rectum and colon to look for suspicious growths and polyps. The camera sends images to a monitor, which allows the doctor to get a good look around.

The procedure itself only takes 30 minutes to an hour, though you must begin preparing for it the night before by taking a preparation designed to flush the colon clean. The cleaner the colon, the better the view and the less likely something will be missed. Dr. Burleson says this is the most difficult part of the procedure, but it's not nearly as bad as it's made out to be. "It only takes a few hours," he says. "By the time you're ready for bed, you're all set."

Before the procedure you'll be given a sedative, so you will not be able to drive yourself to and from the testing site. "You're awake, but with sedation. There is little or no discomfort," he says. "Many patients have told me it wasn't nearly as scary as they expected."

During the procedure the doctor will be looking for any sign of a digestive condition or early signs of cancer. This can include inflammation, bleeding, ulcers, changes in color, and polyps. If a polyp or polyps are found, the doctor may choose to cauterize them or remove them for biopsy.

After the procedure, you will have to rest for an hour or so to allow the sedative to wear off. You may also feel some minor discomfort, such as bloating, gas, and minor bleeding. Because the procedure is invasive it carries risks, the most serious of which is perforation of the intestine. Complications, however, are rare.

The "Other" Colonoscopy

If you're due for a colonoscopy, you've probably heard of and may be wondering about a virtual colonoscopy, which is advertised as being non-invasive and risk-free. A virtual colonoscopy is a CT scan that involves inflating air into the colon and stretching it to get accurate pictures. Its non-invasive nature may make it seem like a breeze, but there are a few downsides:

- It can detect polyps just as a colonoscopy does, but it can't remove them. If an abnormality is detected, you'll have to get a colonoscopy anyway, which doubles your effort and the cost.
- You can't escape the pre-procedure prep. You'll have to go through the same colon-cleansing ritual that is necessary for a traditional colonoscopy.
- Screening should be repeated every five years, instead of 10.
- It exposes you to unnecessary radiation.
- Most insurance companies won't cover it for the above reasons.

Other Screening Options

There are other screening options that are less invasive, less time-consuming, and a lot less costly than colonoscopy. Your doctor may recommend one of these tests if you report vague symptoms and are young and at low risk for colorectal cancer. They are also considered an option for patients who continually ignore their doctor's recommendation to get a screening colonoscopy. Briefly, they are:

Flexible sigmoidoscopy (FSIG). An investigative procedure in which a medical practitioner inserts a pliable tube into the rectum and lower colon. It is an accurate method for seeking the cause of rectal bleeding and requires patient preparation to cleanse the colon. This is more accurate and replaces the procedure called rigid sigmoidoscopy. This test should be repeated every five years.

Double-contrast barium enema. Involves an enema followed by an injection of air and a chalky solution (barium) that shows the outline of the intestines and any abnormalities. This should be repeated every five to 10 years.

Fecal occult blood test (FOBT). A laboratory test of a fecal sample that can detect blood in the stool, but it cannot identify if the blood is coming from a polyp or another source in the body. This test should be repeated yearly.

Fecal immunochemical test (FIT). An at-home test similar to the FOBT, except that it can be purchased over the counter and evaluated by the patient. It also should be repeated yearly.

Diagnosis and Treatment
No matter what test route you take, any abnormality will end in getting a colonoscopy to remove the lesion and a biopsy. Your doctor may then order a CT scan or MRI to determine if the cancer has progressed to other organs. Treatment options depend on the size of the tumor and the stage of the cancer. Surgery is the most common treatment for colorectal cancer.

Know the Symptoms
Generally, colorectal cancer gives no hints of its presence in early stages. As polyps grow, however, they can

bleed or obstruct the intestine. If you experience any of these symptoms, you should see your doctor:

- Rectal bleeding
- Blood in the stool or in the toilet after a bowel movement
- Change in bowel habits
- A change in the size and shape of stools
- Abdominal pain or cramping
- Prolonged constipation

High-Risk Profile
Of all cancers, colorectal is the one most closely aligned with diet and unfavorable lifestyle practices. A high-profile individual might be an overweight, sedentary smoker with a diet high in calories, red meat, and alcohol and low in fiber. People with a history of inflammatory bowel disease are at an increased risk. You also are at increased risk if you have had a parent or sibling with the cancer. People who carry the gene for hereditary nonpolyposis colorectal cancer carry the greatest risk.

ORAL CANCER SCREENING
Screening is part of a routine dental exam, which you should have twice a year but a minimum of once a year.

You may not be aware of it, but every time you to go to the dentist, someone pokes through your mouth looking for signs of cancer. At one time, oral cancer was only a concern in older people with a long history of smoking and/or drinking, but in recent years a new risk factor has developed—exposure to the sexually transmitted human papillomavirus (HPV), the chief cause of cervical cancer.

HPV has created a new paradigm for the disease. Incidence grew 11 percent in just one recent year, largely through detection in men and women in their forties and fifties. The skyrocketing increase has been linked to oral sex with HPV-infected partners—a risk equal to decades of smoking and drinking. The incidence of oral cancer is three times greater than cervical cancer and causes twice as many deaths. Early detection, however, increases survival odds to 80 percent.

A Simple Procedure

Routine screening is nothing more than a visual inspection that lasts about two minutes. Your dentist or a trained associate takes a look at your lips, gums, tongue, roof of the mouth, and the soft tissue inside your cheeks. Generally there are about 10 places inside and around the mouth where precancerous lesions can be found. Dentists are on the lookout for two types of suspicious lesions. One is called oral leukoplakia, which are flat, predominantly white lesions in the lining of the mouth that are not characteristic of another condition, such as a canker sore. The other is oral erythroplakia, which are velvety red, non-removable lesions that harbor early invasive cancer. They can all be seen with the naked eye—even by you—and any qualified dental care practitioner should be able to spot them.

The sharp rise in oral cancer—it is now the sixth most common cancer—has put the American Cancer Society and the American Dental Association on alert that visual screening may no longer be sufficient to reliably spot premalignant cells in high-risk individuals. Your dentists may want to do one of two new screening techniques that are both quick and painless.

One is called a toluidine blue (TB) test, in which the mouth is stained with a blue dye that you then rinse out.

Any stain left behind is the site of suspicious lesions. The other test is called ViziLite, in which the dentist roams through your mouth with a chemiluminescent light. Precancerous and cancerous lesions will reflect the light.

A 2008 study at the University of North Carolina's School of Dentistry found that these tests help increase the odds of early detection of tumors. These new tests can add $35 to $65 to the cost of your annual checkup.

If either of these tests are positive, a sample of tissue will be removed for biopsy.

Diagnosis and Treatment
Only a small fraction of found lesions progress to invasive cancer, which most often is found on the tongue or floor of the mouth. If cancer is found, you will be sent to a specialist for treatment. Treatment depends on the stage of the cancer. Surgery could be required to remove the cancer. HPV-related cancers are usually treated nonsurgically with chemotherapy and radiation.

Prevention: HPV Vaccine
Gardasil is the vaccine currently recommended to protect young girls from getting HPV. Merck, the maker of Gardasil, is seeking government approval to offer the vaccine to boys in hopes of reducing oral cancer in males and other cancers related to the infection.

Know the Symptoms
Cancerous lesions are not painful, but you should be able to see them. Here is what to look for:

• Small ulcer-like sores that feel hard
• Thickening on surfaces of the mouth
• Nodules that feel and look like little bumps

High-Risk Profile

The traditional high-risk candidate is an age 70-plus individual with a lifelong history of smoking, heavy drinking, low consumption of fruit, and perhaps lax dental hygiene practices. Men and women with HPV-infected sex partners are at risk for getting the disease in midlife.

PROSTATE CANCER SCREENING

Your doctor may recommend a yearly PSA blood test starting at age 50.

For a screening credited as being nearly 100 percent effective in detecting early cancer, the simple prostate-specific antigen blood test, commonly called a PSA, brews quite a bit of controversy. Two large population studies made headlines in 2009 for concluding that there is little proof that the test saves lives and only leads to risky and unnecessary treatment in a large number of men—an argument opponents had been making for years.

Nevertheless, the PSA is not going away and for good reason. Prostate cancer is the most common malignancy in American men and the second largest cause of cancer death. The ACS, however, does not recommend routine screening for prostate cancer at this time, but encourages doctors to discuss the option for men beginning at age 50.

Prostate cancer is a malignancy in the walnut-sized gland located at the base of the bladder, which is responsible for controlling urination and semen production. After the PSA test was introduced in 1984, there was a rapid increase in the incidence of prostate cancer, which experts believe was the result of the effectiveness of the PSA in identifying early-stage cancer for which there are no symptoms. There has also been a 30 percent drop in death from the disease, largely due to the PSA and advances in treatment methods.

Detractors of the test claim this drop is small in comparison to the loss of quality of life as a result of getting treatment that they claim may not be necessary. They also say it is difficult to determine whether finding prostate cancer early saves lives because this cancer grows very slowly, meaning it may never be a threat, especially to an older man.

Diagnosis and Treatment

PSA is a protein released by prostate cells. It is not considered a true biomarker for cancer because the test cannot determine if cancer exists; only a biopsy can. High PSA levels suggest that cancer might be present, though this also can be the sign of an enlarged or otherwise inflamed prostate, a condition known as benign prostate hyperplasia, a condition common in men over age 50.

Prior to the PSA, the only detection test for prostate cancer was the digital rectal exam, which doctors still use, even if doing a PSA. In this exam, the doctor gently inserts a gloved finger into the rectum to feel the prostate gland for enlargement or other abnormalities, such as a lump.

An elevated PSA or suspicious physical exam warrants a biopsy. During this procedure, the doctor inserts a transrectal ultrasound probe into the rectum to view the prostate and take a sample of the tissue. The biopsy takes about a half hour and can be done in the doctor's office. Results are usually back in about a week.

If cancer is detected, the results will come back accompanied by a Gleason rating. Prostate cancer contains several types of cells that appear differently under a microscope and are graded on a scale from 2 to 10. The higher the Gleason, the more aggressive the cancer. The Gleason rating, along with other factors, such as age and state of health, determines the treatment options.

Traditionally, surgical removal of the prostate has been the most common treatment, and it is the major reason for the controversy surrounding PSA testing. During a prostatectomy, the surgeon may or may not be able to preserve the neurovascular bundles that are responsible for erection or the urethra that preserves urinary continence. This is where the quality of life issue comes in. Prior to 1980, these nerves were routinely taken to make sure all cancer cells were removed. Today, there are skilled cancer centers that specialize in nerve-sparing surgery, which saves sexual potency. There are also non-surgical methods that attack the tumor with radiation and also spare the nerves. One method, for example, is brachytherapy, in which radioactive seeds are implanted in the prostate to deliver a steady high dose of radiation.

Not every man is a candidate for nerve-sparing surgery or radiation therapy. Generally, the criteria for these treatments are: a tumor in which cells have not escaped the capsule; a PSA level of 10 or less; a Gleason score of 7 or less; and no prior use of medication for erectile dysfunction.

Vague Symptoms

Early-stage prostate cancer has no symptoms. When symptoms do come on, they can be somewhat vague in nature and can vary from man to man. If any of these symptoms persist for two weeks, call your doctor:

- Difficulty urinating
- Weak or interrupted urine flow
- Painful urination
- Frequent urination
- Blood in urine

High-Risk Profile

The cause of prostate cancer is still a mystery, making a high-risk profile difficult to pinpoint. Age, however, is a factor and the cancer typically does not occur until after age 50. African American men have nearly twice the incidence of the disease as Caucasians.

SKIN CANCER SCREENING

The American Cancer Society recommends a cancer-related, whole-body skin checkup by a physician during periodic examinations and self exams starting at age 20.

Skin cancer is the most common type of cancer in the United States. It is also the only cancer that you can actually see, meaning you have it within your power to detect this cancer on your own.

One million new cases of skin cancer are diagnosed in the United States every year. According to current estimates, 40 to 50 percent of Americans will get a cancerous lesion removed at least once by age 65. For the majority, the cancer will be a non-life-threatening basal cell or squamous cell carcinoma. These cancers appear close to the surface of the skin. Melanoma invades deeper into the skin, where it can spread. It accounts for only 3 percent of all skin cancers but can be deadly. If caught early, however, the potential for cure is high.

The ABCDE of Skin Cancer

Looking for early signs of skin cancers is mostly in your own hands. Unless you make an appointment specifically for a full-body skin cancer screening, you should not depend on your primary care physician to give you a thorough skin exam during your routine physical exam. You doctor may want to refer you to a dermatologist for this type of exam. You should also routinely do a self-exam. It's easy. Here's how to go about it:

- Stand naked in front of a full-length mirror in a well-lit room. Look at the front and back of your body in the mirror, then raise your arms and look at your left and right sides. Bend your elbows and look carefully at your fingernails, palms, forearms and upper arms. Look at your thighs and calves and the sides of your legs.
- Turn around and, using a hand-held mirror, look at your back, buttocks, and the backs of your legs. Also look between the buttocks and around the genital area.
- Sit down and closely examine your feet, including the toenails, the soles, and the spaces between the toes.

By checking your skin regularly, about once a month, you will become familiar with what is normal about your skin. Note your birthmarks, moles, blemishes, and freckles—what they look like and how they feel. It's a good idea to write it all down.

Each month, check for anything new, especially a change in size, shape, texture, or color of a mole or tag. Also notice any new area of scaliness, itching, bleeding, tenderness, or pain.

If you detect any change, make an appointment with your doctor for a professional examination. Here is what you, as well as your doctor, should look for. It's called the ABCDE diagnostic system:

- **A**symmetry—the lesion or mole does not look the same all over.
- **B**order—the site has a ragged rather than a smooth edge, which is known as a coastline border.
- **C**olor—the area is multi-colored, often with blue/black pigmentation.
- **D**iameter—usually less than a quarter inch.
- **E**levation—part or all of the lesion is raised.

In some instances, these signs are not always visible to the naked or untrained eye, which is why your doctor may check you out using an instrument that can magnify a blemish 10 times in size.

Basal cell carcinoma is the most common skin cancer. It looks like a small, pink bump or patch and commonly appears on the head or neck, although it can show up anywhere. It is slow-growing and generally does not spread to other parts of the body. If it is not treated, however, it can spread to nearby areas.

Squamous cell carcinoma looks like basal cell, though it is rough and scalier. It also is commonly found on the head or neck but has a tendency to grow on the ears, lips, and the backs of the arms and hands. It is more aggressive than basal cell and can penetrate deeper into the skin.

Melanoma, which forms beneath the outer layers of the skin, usually appears as an irregular brown, black, or red spot. It can also be a mole that begins to change color, size, or shape. It usually appears on the trunk in fair-skinned men and on the lower legs in fair-skinned women. Dark-skinned people tend to get it on the palms of their hands and soles of their feet, where there is less pigment.

Diagnosis and Treatment

Skin cancer diagnosis is made by biopsy. It is a simple procedure in which the doctor excises a sample of tissue for microscopic testing by a pathologist.

There are a variety of treatment options to remove skin tumors, depending on the type of cancer and the thickness of the tumor. It is excised along with a margin of normal skin. Generally, the thicker the tumor, the more likely it is that the cancer has spread. There are several different options for excising basal and squamous cell skin cancers ranging from freezing and destroying the cancerous tissues (called cryosurgery) to laser surgery.

Surgery for melanoma depends on the size and thickness of the tumor. Surgical treatment of small or thin melanoma can consist of excising the tumor and an area of normal tissue surrounding it. Larger melanomas require more extensive surgery and can include removal of lymph nodes in the area of the cancer. If a larger area of skin has to be removed, a skin graft may be required. Radiation therapy may be warranted for all types of skin cancer.

Know the Signs

Symptoms vary from person to person. These symptoms are not always a sign of skin cancer, but warrant a professional evaluation. If one or more of the following doesn't clear up in two weeks, see your doctor:

- A change on the skin, such as a new spot or one that changes in size, shape, or color.
- A sore that doesn't heal.
- A spot or sore that changes in sensation, itchiness, tenderness, or pain.
- A small, smooth, shiny, pale, or waxy lump.
- A firm red lump that may bleed or develops a crust.
- A flat, red spot that is rough, dry, or scaly.

High-Risk Profile

The person most at risk for malignant melanoma is a fair-skinned, red-haired person over age 65, more frequently a man, who lives in the Sun Belt, such as Arizona, and experienced sunburns as a child. In men, melanoma most often occurs on the trunk and shoulder of the body, followed by the upper arms and face. In women, the most common site is the lower legs, followed by the arms.

In both men and women under age 50, the primary site for melanoma is on the back. After age 50, it occurs on all areas exposed to the sun, often the face.

ENDOMETRIAL (UTERINE) CANCER DETECTION

There are currently no effective screening tests to detect this cancer. Women past menopause should continue to have annual pelvic exams that may be able to detect signs of the disease.

Endometrial cancer, a malignancy of the lining of the uterus, is the most common cancer of the female reproductive system. It is considered a disease that strikes older women. It is rare in women under age 45 and more than half the cases are diagnosed in women between the ages of 55 and 70. The cause of endometrial cancer is not known and the disease is not fully understood, but doctors believe it is linked to a lifetime exposure to high levels of the female hormone estrogen that are not counterbalanced by progesterone.

Looking for Cancer

Even though there is no screening to detect the disease at a precancerous stage, it can be detected at the earliest possible stage if you keep up with your annual gynecological exam and Pap tests, especially after menopause. A Pap test can sometimes detect endometrial changes, but it is not considered an effective test for diagnosing the cancer. During your annual exam, your doctor will ask you if you've had any abnormal vaginal bleeding, which is often the sign of uterine trouble in older women.

If you have bleeding or the pelvic exam raises any suspicions, your doctor will likely schedule a transvaginal ultrasound, a procedure in which an instrument is inserted into the vagina to check for thickness of the endometrium, a possible sign of cancer. If this occurs, a biopsy will follow.

A uterine biopsy is a simple procedure in which a doctor removes a sample of tissue from the uterine lining. It can be done in the doctor's office. In some cases, however, a woman may need to have a more invasive procedure called dilation and curettage, commonly known as a D&C. This is usually done as same-day surgery with anesthesia in a hospital. A pathologist will examine the biopsy sample for signs of cancer. A biopsy can cause cramps and some bleeding afterward.

Treatment depends on the stage of the cancer, but usually involves hysterectomy (removal of the uterus) and sometimes radiation therapy. Treatment with hormone therapy to prevent estrogen from feeding tumor cells is sometimes recommended.

Endometrial cancer is highly curable, with the rate around 90 percent.

Know the Symptoms

Bleeding is not a normal part of menopause and warrants a visit to the doctor. Call your gynecologist for an appointment if you experience any of these symptoms:

- Abnormal bleeding after menopause
- Difficult or painful urination
- Painful intercourse
- Pelvic pain

High-Risk Profile

Childless, overweight, older women who started menstruating before age 12 and started menopause after age 55 are most at risk. Diabetes, high blood pressure, a high-fat diet, and hormone replacement therapy add to the risk. Other risk factors include taking Tamoxifen for treatment or prevention of breast cancer and a history of endometrial hyperplasia, which is a thickening of the uterine lining. Women who carry the gene for hereditary nonpolysis colorectal cancer (HNPCC), which can only be found through genetic testing, have a 40 percent increased risk for endometrial cancer.

LUNG CANCER DETECTION

Currently, there is no effective test to detect lung cancer at an early stage.

It's a sad irony that the most prevalent cancer killer would be a rare cancer if tobacco and smoking didn't exist. It's even sadder that there is no effective way to screen for lung cancer before a person experiences symptoms. Lung cancer is the result of cells multiplying uncontrollably in the lungs, damaging surrounding tissue and interfering with the normal function of the lung. It tends to spread (metastasize) to other parts of the body very early in its course, making it a challenge to treat. Due to this and the lack of early warning signs, lung cancer has one of the poorest survival rates of all cancers.

Diagnosis and Treatment

Early-forming tumors in the lung are not always visible on X-ray. A sputum cytology test, which analyzes coughed-up mucus, can detect the presence of a tumor. If you have been a longtime smoker, your doctor can give you this test even if you have no symptoms. It's a noninvasive way to help detect the cancer in its early stages.

If you already have symptoms, your doctor might opt to do a bronchoscopy, a procedure in which a thin flexible tube with a tiny camera is inserted through the nose or mouth and down into the lungs. During this procedure, sample tissue can be taken for biopsy.

There are several types of lung cancers and treatment options depend on knowing the type and stage of the cancer. There are a variety of different tests that can help doctors decide the course of treatment, including a CAT scan, which takes computerized pictures of the lungs, and Positron Emission Tomography (PET), a special type of scanner that contains a radioactive atom that is injected into a vein to spot abnormal cells.

The standard surgery for lung cancer includes removal of the lobe of the lung in which the tumor resides (lobectomy) and dissection and removal of the lymph nodes. However, advances in minimally invasive surgery are improving treatment outcomes for many people with lung cancer. For advanced lung cancer, surgery is often not an option. In this case, the course of treatment is radiation or radiation combined with chemotherapy.

Different Tumor, Different Symptoms

A troubling aspect of lung cancer is that symptoms vary depending on the location and size of the tumor and how far it has spread. Any number of these symptoms could be a sign of lung cancer. If you are a smoker or at high risk for any other reason, see your doctor if you experience any of the following:

- Persistent cough
- Labored breathing
- Chest pain
- Wheezing
- Persistent hoarseness
- Fatigue
- Loss of appetite
- Weight loss

High-Risk Profile

Smoking is the cause of an estimated 90 percent of lung cancer cases. It usually results after decades of smoking. Other causes include exposure to secondhand smoke, asbestos, radon, and other harmful pollutants. People with chronic lung disease are at higher risk for lung cancer.

OVARIAN CANCER DETECTION

There is currently no effective screening test to detect this cancer early.

The cause of ovarian cancer is somewhat of a mystery, which is why there currently is no effective method for prevention or early detection. Unfortunately, the disease has no telling set of symptoms. Because the symptoms are vague, diagnosis is difficult and often does not occur until late stages of malignancy. Of the 25 percent that are discovered early, however, the five-year survival rate is more than 90 percent.

Not all ovarian tumors are malignant. There are some 30 different types of ovarian tumors, some of which are benign. About 90 percent of tumors are epithelial ovarian cancer, meaning that the tumor is in the tissue that covers the outside of the ovary. Risk for this type of tumor increases with age and most often occurs past 60, although it can develop at any age.

Detection and Treatment

The first indication of ovarian cancer is often made during a pelvic exam when the doctor palpitates the lower abdomen while examining the vagina to feel for a mass on either side of the uterus.

A doctor who suspects ovarian cancer or wants to rule it out may want to do a transvaginal ultrasound or a blood test or both. The ultrasound receives echoes that bounce off the ovaries, creating images that the doctor can view on a small screen. A radiologist interprets the results. Another test is a blood sample that measures the level of a protein called CA-125.

The only way to confirm a diagnosis is through biopsy, which in this case is a surgical procedure done in the hospital. During the surgery, a pathologist will read the results, which could lead to immediate invasive surgery to remove the tumor and affected organs.

In addition to surgery, chemotherapy is usually recommended. Radiation is seldom used for ovarian cancer.

THE TALCUM SCARE

In the days before asbestos became a known carcinogen, talcum powder was a common everyday
hygienic product that mothers routinely used to
freshen a baby's bottom. Some women also put it
in their panties to freshen the genital area.

Talc, the mineral used to make the powder,
contains minute particles of naturally occurring
asbestos. As a result of its cancer connection, talcum powder became suspect as a cause of several
types of cancer, including lung and ovarian cancers. All have been ruled out, except for ovarian
cancer, though the evidence is still inconclusive.

Talcum powder, however, is no longer a threat
and federal laws have required that all powders
be free of asbestos since the mid-1970s.

Know the Symptoms

The symptoms of ovarian cancer are so subtle that it is
easy to dismiss them as typical gastrointestinal upset
or part of aging. Contact your doctor if you experience
the following:

- Abdominal discomfort, such as indigestion, pres-
  sure, cramps or gas
- Bloating or a sense of fullness even after a light
  meal
- Unexplainable weight loss or weight gain
- Fatigue
- Loss of appetite

High-Risk Profile

The high-risk profile is an overweight childless woman over age 50 or 60 who has a family history of ovarian cancer and personal history of breast or colon cancer. Taking hormone replacement therapy (HRT) or fertility drugs may also increase the risk.

GENETIC TESTING

It's well known that cancer can run in the family. It's also well established that most people who have cancer in the family will never get it themselves. Why this happens is still a mystery and thousands of scientists around the world are trying to solve it.

One of the most active areas of cancer research involves looking for genes that can set off the cellular cartwheels that lead to cancer. The most advanced progress to date is the isolation of genes that are markers for breast, colorectal, endometrial, and ovarian cancers. BRCA-1 and BRCA-2 are known biomarkers for breast and ovarian cancers, and MLH-1 and MLH-2 are markers for colon and endometrial cancer. Having a cancer gene is no guarantee that you will get the cancer, but it raises the odds significantly.

There are obvious pros and cons involved in making the decision to find out if you possess one of these genes. The American Society of Clinical Oncology recommends that genetic testing be done only under these circumstances, which you should review with your doctor.

- You have personal or family history that your doctor agrees is suggestive of a genetic susceptibility.
- There is a genetic test for the cancer of your concern that is considered reliable and can be adequately interpreted.

- You are fully aware of the consequences of a positive diagnosis.
- You engage in professional psychological counseling to help you manage the decision you may have to make by knowing you possess the gene. This can include surgical intervention and other quality-of-life tradeoffs versus the probably added years to your life.

CHAPTER 4

Foods That Help Fight Cancer

The best foods on Earth that are protective against cancer are those kissed by the sun. The biochemical process (called photosynthesis) that helps plant food grow injects them with an abundance of precious nutrients, enriching the body in a variety of special ways.

These are not just the vitamins and minerals that we strive to get daily to sustain healthy organs and support everyday life. Plant foods also possess other naturally occurring nutrients, called phytochemicals, with the unique ability to protect cells against the corrosive processes that weaken the immune system and make you more vulnerable to cancer-causing substances.

Phytochemicals (or phytonutrients) are an umbrella term for scores of natural chemicals with hundreds of subclasses that researchers have found are significant to feeling good and living a robust life. In short, phytochemicals help prevent many diseases and one of them is cancer.

Research shows that some have a special ability to stop the inflammatory processes that set cells off on a cancerous direction. Many of them act as powerful antioxidants that help boost the cancer-fighting strength of certain vitamins and minerals and help them work even harder to defend the body. Some of these nutrients have been found to help stop tumor growth and even make tumors disappear.

Scientists have uncovered thousands of these micronutrients and believe there are thousands more yet to be discovered. This is why making good food choices is so important in living an anti-cancer lifestyle. Diet is possibly the strongest defense we have in helping to reduce our risk of getting cancer. Studies indicate that if everyone ate a healthy anti-cancer diet high in antioxidant fruits and vegetables and limited in animal food, the incidence of cancer would drop an estimated 30 percent.

THE CASE FOR FRUITS AND VEGETABLES

Nature's foods—the fruits and vegetables that grow on trees and vines—are the backbone of an anti-cancer diet. The American Cancer Society (ACS) recommends that we eat a minimum of four or five servings a day. Unfortunately, we don't even get close. According to recent surveys, only 32.6 percent of American adults said they eat two or more servings of fruit a day, and even fewer said they eat three or more servings of vegetables a day.

Yet, there is overwhelming evidence illustrating the importance of fruits and vegetables in the daily diet. Thousands of studies over decades of research show that as consumption of fruits and vegetables goes up, cancer risk comes down. For example:

- Numerous studies indicate that colorectal cancer is highest in people who eat a high-fat diet and lowest in those who eat a nutrient-dense, high-fiber diet rich in fruits and vegetables.

- One study specifically showed that eating 17 ounces of fruit and vegetables a day reduces the risk of cancers of the digestive tract by 25 to 50 percent.
- Cruciferous vegetables, such as broccoli, cauliflower, and cabbage, have been shown to lower the risk of breast, bladder, colorectal, endometrial, lung, prostate, and ovarian cancers.
- Dozens of studies in Italy found that people who eat more fruit than vegetables have a lower incidence of cancers affecting the lower digestive tract; people who eat more vegetables than fruit have a lower incidence of cancers of the upper digestive tract, stomach, and urinary tract.
- Major, long-term studies following the dietary habits of 77,283 nurses and 47,778 doctors in the United States show that consuming fruits and vegetables has a protective effect against secondhand smoke.
- Polish researchers found that when vegetables are eaten with grilled meat—a ratio of more vegetables than meat—the body does not absorb polycyclic aromatic hydrocarbons (PAHs), toxic substances that are produced on meat grilled at a high temperature. The researchers theorize that the vegetables have the ability to neutralize the toxic substances.
- Though findings have been inconsistent, a diet excessively rich in starchy foods—mainly beans, flour products and simple sugars—and low in fruits and vegetables may be associated with an increased risk of stomach cancer.

An estimated 25,000 phytonutrients have been identified that scientists believe have potential to fight various cancers. This means you can feel assured that *all* fruits and vegetables, including the vast array of natural whole grains, contain some of them. Thousands of studies have been conducted looking for the foods that are the best sources of anti-cancer nutrients. This chapter is an A-to-Z guide to 40 foods that have been proven to be among the most potent cancer fighters and includes tips on how to buy these foods and prepare them in ways that are both tasty and preserve their nutritional value.

APPLES

An apple a day may keep the doctor away, but three apples a day can help keep the oncologist away.

Research at Cornell University has found that apples—and specifically apple peel—contain powerful substances called phenols and flavonoids that can help inhibit the deadliest types of **breast cancer**.

In the Cornell studies, rats were exposed to the particular type of tumor that is the main cause of death among breast cancer patients as well as test animals. For 24 weeks the rats were fed daily doses of fresh apple extracts—the equivalent of eating one, three, or six apples a day in humans. Another group was given no apples.

Tumor formation was inhibited in more than 50 percent of the animals, but was most effective in those fed the most apple extract. Cancer developed in 57 percent of the rats fed the equivalent of one apple a day, 50 percent in those given the medium dose, and in only 23 percent given the highest dose. They also found that the nutrients in apples can block breast cells from mutating into malignant tumors.

The researchers believe the phenol and flavonoid makeup in apples interrupts and turns off the chemi-

ANTI-CANCER DIET GUIDELINES

- Eat four to five servings, or a minimum of 14 ounces of fruits and vegetables, a day.
- Eat no more than 3 ounces of red meat a day.
- Eat processed meats, such as sausage and charcuterie, only occasionally.
- Consume salty and cured foods only occasionally.
- Do not drink liquids or eat foods that are scalding hot.
- Drink alcohol in moderation and preferably at mealtime.
- Avoid simple carbohydrates and other foods with a high glycemic index as much as possible.
- Eat grilled meats, chicken, and fish in moderation and always avoid charring.
- Eat a helping of cruciferous vegetables, such as broccoli, cabbage, and kale, every day or as much as possible.
- Avoid foods that are not 100 percent natural. This includes processed and junk foods and anything containing additives, chemicals, and dyes.
- Avoid foods that have been treated with chemicals, sprays, or wax.
- Steer clear of trans fats. This includes anything with the words "hydrogenated" or "partially hydrogenated."

cal pathway of breast cancer cells. Apples contain the highest levels of phenols and flavonoids among the top 25 most consumed fruits.

"We not only observed that the treated animals had

fewer tumors, but the tumors were smaller, less malignant and grew more slowly compared with the tumors in the untreated rats," said Rui Hai Liu, Cornell associate professor of food science and a member of Cornell's Institute for Comparative and Environmental Toxicology.

"These studies add to the growing evidence that increased consumption of fruits and vegetables, including apples, would provide consumers with more phenolics, which are proving to have important health benefits," said Liu. "I would encourage consumers to eat more and a wide variety of fruits and vegetables daily."

Other research in test animals has found apples to be protective against other cancers as well, including **skin, colon,** and **lung cancers.**

In the Kitchen with Apples

Eating an apple or two a day is easy to do because an apple's protective effects can be found in all its forms—juice, cider, sauce, butter, and as a dried fruit. And, of course, you can't beat the simple pleasure of eating an apple out of hand. Make sure to eat the skin as well, because of its special nutrient content.

Apples come in hundreds of varieties, both sweet and tart, and are available year round. They can keep for months as long as you buy them "sound," meaning they should be firm and richly colored without any bruising. They are best kept in a cool place where air can circulate around them. Here are a few ideas on different ways to enjoy apples:

• Ancient Romans ate diced pork and apples. You can do the same thing by adding diced or sliced apples to pork and vegetable stir-fries.

- Make apple pie more nutritious by eating it British style, with only a crust on top.
- Dice apples into sauerkraut or baked red cabbage.
- Add them to fruit salads and green salads. You can keep them from turning brown after slicing by putting them in water with a tablespoon or two of lemon juice.
- Serve apple slices instead of crackers on a cheese tray.

AVOCADOS

When you see an avocado, does your mind think *sinfully delicious*? Well, then, it's time to change your mindset, because the buttery, rich yellow-green flesh of the avocado is mighty powerful when it comes to fighting tumors.

An analysis of several studies found that the avocado contains a wide array of phytochemicals that individually and selectively target tumors for extinction. "These studies suggest that individual and combinations of phytochemicals from the avocado fruit may offer an advantageous dietary strategy in cancer prevention," reported researchers from Ohio State University, who analyzed the research.

The Ohio State researchers believe the fruit contains a variety of nutrients that individually or in concert have the ability to track the free radical pathways of precancerous and cancerous cells and kill them without causing any damage to healthy cells. They found avocado to be particularly effective against **oral cancer.**

The researchers didn't say what amount of avocado is necessary to keep the oral cavity healthy, but you'll give your taste buds extra pleasure by including them in your diet as much as possible. Avocados are also a rich source of oleic acid, a monounsaturated fat—known as "the good fat." They also contain other anti-cancer nutrients, including fiber, folate, and vitamin C.

In a separate study at UCLA, researchers found the nutrients in avocados can help fight **prostate cancer.**

In the Kitchen with Avocado

There are several varieties of avocados, but go for Haas, if possible, because this is the fruit that was used in the scientific studies and is believed to have the highest concentration of anti-cancer nutrients.

Avocados ripen off the tree, so you usually need to buy them in advance of using. You'll know the fruit is ripe when the flesh gives a little when you press it, especially at the stem end. They can ripen in the refrigerator, but if you're in a hurry, you can keep them out at room temperature. Depending on how long it's been off the tree, an avocado can take one to two weeks to ripen.

Guacamole is the most famous avocado dish. Feel free to dig in, because every ingredient in guacamole—avocado, chili pepper, onion, tomato, and lemon juice—is on the anti-cancer diet. To keep it totally healthy, serve with pita wedges instead of chips.

There are many ways to serve avocados and, because of their brilliant color, they always make a great presentation. Here are some ideas:

- Slice an avocado in half, scoop out the stone, and scoop in shrimp, crab, lobster, or chicken salad.
- Stack slices of avocado with turkey on whole grain bread. Add some sprouts for crunch.
- Dice it and add it to homemade or store-bought salsa. It is a natural with tomatoes.

- Serve it sliced aside or on top of a grilled burger to help neutralize potentially cancer-causing substances that accumulate in grilled meats. Add a tomato as well.
- Mash it and eat it on warmed whole-grain bread as a snack or appetizer.
- Add slices of avocado and papaya to a salad for a light, nutritious luncheon.
- Take advantage of nutritious avocado oil as an alternative to canola or olive oil in dressings and sautés.

BEANS

Mexican food isn't noted for being healthy, but Mexico and South America are home to an important crop that often gets overlooked as an important cancer fighter—the common bean.

Two different research groups in Mexico, where beans are the most important food next to corn, found that 62 varieties of beans from south of the border contain the same variety of phytonutrients with cancer-fighting activity that have been so well-studied in vegetables. Both cultivated and wild beans possess these nutrients, but wild varieties are by far the richest. They can be spotted by their pigmented coat and come in a variety of colors, including white, pink, yellow, red, and black.

Researchers at Michigan State University put Mexican beans to the **colon cancer** test by feeding laboratory rats a diet consisting of 75 percent black beans or 75 percent navy beans for four weeks. In week five they induced the rats with colon cancer-causing substances. After 31 weeks, only 9 percent of the rats fed black beans and 14 percent fed navy beans developed colon cancer. This was significantly lower than the 36 percent tumor rate in the rats that were not fed beans. The researchers concluded that "eating black beans and navy beans significantly lowered colon cancer incidence and multiplicity."

In the Kitchen with Beans

Shopping for exotic beans can be great fun. Look for them in markets that cater to Mexican or South American communities or restaurants. When checking the bins, look for plump, glossy beans that are not withered. Store them, without washing, in a bag or container in a cool place.

When you're ready to use them, spread them out on a large plate and separate out any debris. Toss out any damaged beans. Wash them in a colander under cool running water.

Dried beans need to be soaked overnight or for at least eight hours. Before using them in your recipe, drain and rinse well one more time. Cook the beans on the stovetop or in a pressure cooker.

There are an infinite number of ways to feature beans including in soups, chili, burritos and as salad. They pair well with tomatoes, onions, and salsa and are a great side dish with burgers or summer barbecue fare. If you're short on time, buy them canned. Just make sure to rinse them to get rid of excess salt.

BERRIES

When it comes to anti-cancer foods, you can't do much better than a bowl full of berries.

For being so tiny and fragile, berries—blueberries, cranberries, strawberries, black raspberries, blackberries, red raspberries—are a fortress of antioxidant and anti-inflammatory nutrients with a potent ability to help stop the initiation and progression of cancerous tumors at the cellular level.

Berries contain the most powerful cancer-fighting vitamins—A, C, E, and folic acid—and minerals—calcium and selenium. They are also a powerhouse of polyphenols, including quercitin, ellagic acid, and a broad spectrum of unique nutrients called anthocyanins that accumulate in their sun-kissed skin.

In more than a dozen animal and human studies conducted at Ohio State University in Columbus, scientists found berries to be potent against a variety of cancers and, in most instances, the black raspberry appeared to be the mightiest of them all. In fact, the skin of the black raspberry is so rich (it possesses four major types of anthocyanins) that one animal study found it was strong enough to show a protective effect against the ultraviolet rays of the sun that can lead to **skin cancer**. In another study in rats, the same researchers found that powders made from both black raspberries, strawberries, blackberries, and blueberries can help prevent **esophageal cancer**. Black raspberry powder was even more powerful against **colon cancer**. It helped slow the growth rate of pre-malignant polyps that lead to cancer, thus reducing the risk of getting colon cancer by 80 percent. And in human studies, a black raspberry gel was shown to resolve suspicious lesions in the mouths of 17 people at risk for **oral cancer**.

Researchers believe the abundance of cancer-defensive nutrients in berries works by inhibiting carcinogen-induced damage to cell DNA and by reducing the growth of premalignant cells and stimulating these cells to die. They also markedly reduce inflammation.

"Although we have principally worked with black

raspberries, it looks like many other berry types also appear to be protective against cancer," said Gary D. Stoner, Ph.D., a principal researcher at Ohio State's Comprehensive Cancer Center, where much of the berry research is being done. "It would benefit anyone to eat a few helpings of fresh berries every week."

In the Kitchen with Berries

Most people find no problem getting their fair share of berries, especially during the summer when fresh berries are at their best and cheapest. There's no need to shy away from frozen varieties, however. Dr. Stoner says frozen berries retain their nutritional value for up to a year.

Unfortunately, the best anti-cancer berry is the hardest to find. The large blackberries you customarily see in the market are not black raspberries. Black raspberries are the same size as red raspberries and do not grow in the wild to the extent of blackberries. They are more difficult to grow and not as readily available in the supermarket. So when you see them, make sure to take advantage of their goodness and healing potential. (You can get black raspberry as a supplement. For more information see page 157).

When buying fresh berries, check that they are free of blemishes and their color is bright and brilliant. Refrigerate them, unwashed, in an uncovered container lined with paper towels to absorb the moisture. They will stay fresh for several days. Wash and bring them to room temperature before using.

Berries' culinary possibilities are almost endless. Other than eating them out of hand, here are some ideas:

- Sprinkle them over your morning cereal or add them to creamy or frozen yogurt.
- Make a dessert topping by putting 2 cups of fresh

or frozen berries in a food processor with a cup of confectioner's sugar and 2 tablespoons of lemon juice. If you're using raspberries or mixing berries, add a tablespoon of Chambord.

• For a pancake topping, poach two cups of fresh or frozen berries in half a cup of water and half a cup of brown sugar. Simmer, covered, for about 15 minutes. You can also use this topping on frozen yogurt, pie, or in a parfait.

• Make a blueberry or raspberry sauce to accent poultry or game by combining 2 cups of berries, ¼ cup orange juice, ½ cup sugar, 1 tablespoon lime juice and a pinch of cinnamon and cloves in a saucepan and heat until the berries pop.

BROCCOLI

Broccoli is the most esteemed member of the *Brassica* family, a group of low-calorie, intensely flavored vegetables with a special ability to stop the oxidation process that leads to cancer. *Brassica*, also known as cruciferous vegetables, are believed to possess more anti-tumor activity than any other vegetable. "There is ever-increasing evidence that a high consumption of *Brassica* vegetables may reduce the risk of several types of cancer," says Robert Verpoorte, a pharmacologist and plant researcher from the Netherlands.

Numerous animal and human studies indicate that broccoli is the most potent *Brassica* of all. It contains at least 10 compounds with well-known cancer-fighting activity, including beta-carotene, vitamin C, lutein, and quercetin. It's also a rare rich source of folic acid and it possesses more phenols, a type of phytochemical that fights cancer, than any other food in the plant kingdom.

What's possibly most unique about broccoli as a

cancer-fighting vegetable, however, is its ability to accumulate and pool selenium, a nutrient known to have cancer-preventive action, in a way that is protective against **breast** and **colon cancers**.

Broccoli is a rich source of selenium and its selenium content is also uncharacteristically potent. Researchers at the Grand Forks Human Nutrition Center in North Dakota found that selenium-rich broccoli is more protective as a cancer preventive than selenium alone.

Researchers in Buffalo tested its effectiveness in an experiment that included more than 1,500 women in Erie and Niagara counties in New York State, an area with a high incidence of breast cancer. They found that consuming broccoli on a regular basis appeared to reduce the risk of getting breast cancer prior to menopause, though it did not have the same protective effect on post-menopausal women.

In Italy, researchers put 20 young and healthy smokers and non-smokers on a broccoli-rich diet for 10 days and found that eating broccoli daily had an extra-protective effect against DNA damage caused by smoking.

Broccoli and Tomatoes: A Powerful Prostate-protecting Team
Broccoli, as do other cruciferous vegetables, contains at least four classes of phytonutrients that help fight cancer, including indoles that are believed to be protective against **prostate cancer**. Tomatoes contain a variety of antioxidant vitamins plus lycopene, a nutrient well known for being a potent prostate protector. With two nutrients so loaded with cancer-preventive antioxidants, researchers in Illinois and Ohio wondered how they would come out in a head-to-head match against prostate cancer.

In the experiment, the researchers fed powdered extracts of broccoli and tomatoes to test rats in three combinations. One team of rats was fed a diet containing 10 percent broccoli, another team was fed a diet containing 10 percent tomatoes, and a third team was fed a diet containing 5 percent broccoli and 5 percent tomatoes. Two other teams were also enlisted in the experiment, with each being fed a different dosage of supplemental lycopene. One month into the diet, the rats were implanted with prostate tumors. After 22 months, the scientists examined their tumor growth.

They found that all five combinations reduced the size of the tumors, but the tomatoes and broccoli together had the greatest impact, shrinking the tumors by an average of 52 percent. Broccoli alone reduced tumor size by 42 percent compared to tomatoes alone at 34 percent. The lycopene supplement produced an 18 percent reduction at the larger dose and a 7 percent reduction at the smaller dose.

The fact that the two foods were more powerful as a team came as no surprise to the researchers—adding to the proof that food may be more powerful than a single nutrient when it comes to preventing disease.

In human terms, the rats were fed the equivalent of 4 cups of broccoli a day and 2½ cups of fresh tomatoes or 1 cup of tomato sauce.

In the Kitchen with Broccoli

Buy broccoli with heads that are dark green with a purple or blue hue. Heads that are turning yellow indicate they are beyond their peak. Refrigerate in an open plastic bag for up to three days.

Enzymes in broccoli activate the nutritional content when it is cut or sliced, so don't cut into broccoli until just before you are ready to use it. Also, nutritional content is compromised with cooking, so it is best to eat it raw or cook it briefly. Broccoli's flavor is so intense it does not require more than a simple steam for 5 minutes, or stir-fry for a few minutes with olive oil. Boiling and microwaving reduces nutritional content 30 to 50 percent.

Broccoli is such a potent cancer fighter, try to eat it as much as possible—daily if you can. To do that, you'll want a little variety. Here are some ideas:

- Cut broccoli into tiny florets and add to your daily salad. Make sure the salad also has tomatoes, so you get the combination protection. Serve it with yogurt dressing or a sesame ginger vinaigrette.
- Snip it into tomato soup as it comes to a simmer and let it cook 2 minutes before serving.
- Eat it raw as a snack with peanut dipping sauce.
- Steam lightly and sprinkle on top of pizza.
- Sauté it in olive oil with garlic, onions, and tomatoes.
- Put it in tomato sauce and serve over pasta.
- Combine it with cheese for a morning omelet.

BROCCOLI SPROUTS

Talk about going green! Broccoli sprouts are a superhero when it comes to defending your airways from secondhand smoke, air pollution, and other invisible airborne menaces.

Broccoli sprouts are the vegetable kingdom's richest source of sulforaphane, a special antioxidant that acts as a filter to your lungs. Researchers at UCLA wanted to find out just how powerful sulforaphane is, so they fed a group of allergy-prone people a big helping of broccoli sprouts in the great outdoors. A similar group was given bean sprouts, which contains no sulforaphane,

under the same conditions. They found that sulforaphane boosted the presence of protective antioxidant
enzymes in the nasal passages two to threefold, blocking pollen and pollutants from getting to the lung. There
was no change in the enzymes in the nasal passages of
the bean sprouts eaters.

The researchers concluded that eating broccoli sprouts
is a powerful ally in protecting the airways and could
be a beneficial shield against **lung** and **esophageal
cancers**. The amount of broccoli sprouts it took to induce this positive reaction was 7 ounces.

Suforaphane's detoxifying action stretches all the way
to the sun. While replenishing lotion can help soothe
skin after too much time in the sun, a helping of broccoli sprouts can actually help reduce the damage occurring deep in the skin's cells.

In one study, scientists exposed test animals to harmful ultraviolet light equal to sunbathing on the beach on
a clear summer day. The animals took a sunbath twice
a week for 20 weeks. Five nights a week, the researchers soothed tiny mouse backs with a topical solution
containing broccoli extract. They found the extract
helped counteract the damage to skin cells that can lead
to **skin cancer**.

Broccoli sprouts should also be on your plate if
you're ill as a result of the *Helicobacter pylori* bacteria.
H. pylori is a well-known cause of ulcers, but it can also
lead to **stomach cancer**. Several studies have found that
sulforaphane extract from broccoli sprouts had the power
to kill human *H. pylori*.

Broccoli's potential as a preventive against *H. pylori*,
of course, would pique the interest of researchers in Japan, where the rate of stomach cancer is the highest in
the world. Japanese doctors fed hospitalized patients infected with the bacterium 3.5 ounces of broccoli a day

and found it speeded up the healing process. Researchers in Hawaii, where the incidence of stomach cancer is also high, did a similar experiment and found that "intake of vegetables, especially cruciferous vegetables, had a stronger protective effect" against stomach cancer.

A few ounces a day are enough to elevate the body's protective enzymes.

In the Kitchen with Broccoli Sprouts

You can find fresh broccoli sprouts at specialty markets and at many supermarkets in major areas. Make sure to eat them soon after buying because they get limp in a few days.

Use them as you would other sprouts. They make sandwiches crunchy and add extra flavor to everyday salads. They can be sautéed or stir-fried, but should only be in the pan for 20 to 30 seconds.

BRUSSELS SPROUTS

Brussels sprouts may never win an award as the world's favorite vegetable, but they deserve a place of honor as a loyal cancer fighter.

Like other members of the cruciferous family, Brussels sprouts possess a number of cancer-fighting substances, but their unique contribution comes from their ability to neutralize the toxic effects of carcinogens that lead to **colon** and **lung cancers.** This ability comes from its abundance of glucosinolate, a phytochemical that helps detoxify harmful substances in the liver. All crucifers are rich in glucosinolates, but the tiny deep green orbs contain about three times more than a big head of red and green cabbage.

In one experiment, researchers implanted lab rats with carcinogens known to cause precancerous lesions in the liver and colon. They then fed one group water mixed with Brussels sprout juice; another group was fed water spiked with red cabbage juice. Both juices were effective at reducing the number of precancerous lesions in the liver and colon, but the Brussels sprouts juice was far more effective, reducing the development of precancerous colon polyps by around 50 percent and diminishing the size of precancerous lesions in the liver by an outstanding 91 percent.

Brussels sprouts also proved to be equally effective at diminishing the toxic effects of the carcinogens in tobacco that lead to **lung cancer**. Researchers in the Netherlands tested the blood of 10 smokers for residual signs of tobacco toxins. They then divided the group in two. One group ate 10.5 ounces of Brussels sprouts a day, while the other group was instructed not to eat any cruciferous vegetables. After three weeks, the Brussels sprouts eaters showed a 28 percent reduction in DNA damage compared to the smokers who didn't eat any.

In the Kitchen with Brussels Sprouts

Indeed, not everyone is a fan of Brussels sprouts. A survey at Baruch College in New York City found that only 10 percent of students admitted to liking them but perhaps that's because they may never have had them prepared the right way! Brussels sprouts have a robust, rich flavor, but they can taste bitter if not properly prepared.

Young sprouts have the sweetest taste. At certain times of the year, you can find Brussels sprouts at market still attached to their stalks. Most times, you'll find them loose or in a box. Choose smaller heads over larger. Look for firm compact heads that are heavy for their size. Brussels sprouts should be used within three days of purchase or they will start to taste bitter.

Before cooking, peel off the loose outer leaves. If you are cooking them whole, cut an X into the stem. However, they will cook more evenly if you cut them in half. Here are a few cooking ideas:

- Try them the way the Belgians like them— sautéed with peeled chestnuts. Brown shallots in olive oil, add canned chestnuts, cover halfway with beef broth, add thyme and parsley, cover, and cook about 15 minutes. If using fresh chestnuts, bake until the chestnuts are soft.
- Make Brussels sprouts "French fries." Cut the sprouts in half and put them in a small bowl. Add 1–2 tablespoons of olive oil and toss to coat. Put the sprouts on a baking sheet and bake at 375°F preheated for 20 minutes or until crisp and crunchy.

CABBAGE

If you are among the many people who don't like the odor of cooked cabbage lingering in the kitchen, then take advantage of this vegetable in the raw. Eating just three servings of raw cabbage a month can reduce the risk of **bladder cancer** by 40 percent. Cole slaw and salad lovers eat it more often than that!

Cabbage's bladder-protecting action comes from compounds called isothiocyanates, or ITCs. ITCs are present in all cruciferous vegetables, but they start to dissipate as soon as the vegetable hits the heat. That's what makes cabbage so special. It is a natural for eating in the raw.

For years, researchers didn't think ITCs had much healing power, because experiments linking them to cancer prevention showed inconsistent results. That was until 2007, when researchers at Roswell Park Cancer Center in Buffalo discovered a difference in the rate of bladder cancer among people who ate raw and cooked cruciferous vegetables. Other studies have also linked ITCs to a reduced incidence of **breast**, **lung**, and **pancreatic** cancer.

Cabbage has more going for it than just ITCs. Cabbage contains dozens of other cancer-fighting phytochemicals that are not destroyed by cooking. Cooking, however, does not destroy all of cabbage's nutritional action. Studies in countries where large amounts of cabbage are consumed, such as East Germany and Poland, have a lower incidence of **stomach cancer** and cancers of the **digestive tract**.

In the Kitchen with Cabbage

Cancer-fighting substances can be found in all white, red, and Chinese cabbages. Among the three, red cabbage is most frequently eaten raw. The red outer shell is a sign that it contains anthocyanins, a special cancer-fighting pigment more common in fruit. When boiled in water, red cabbage will lose its color, so it is best to eat it in its natural state.

You can eat cabbage and still retain an ample amount of ITCs by grilling it. Lightly brush the cabbage leaves with Caesar salad dressing or light olive oil. Grill for a minute or two on each side.

To make a red cabbage slaw, sauté one head of sliced cabbage and a small red onion, thinly sliced, in a tablespoon of olive oil for one minute. Transfer to a bowl. Combine 3 tablespoons each of balsamic vinegar and brown sugar and a half teaspoon of allspice and pour it over the cabbage. Let it sit in the refrigerator for about a day befor eating.

CANOLA OIL

What does a bottle of canola oil have in common with cabbage? A whole lot, it turns out. Canola is a vegetable oil that also goes by a lesser-known name, rapeseed oil, and rape is a member of the cancer-fighting cruciferous family—and a high-ranking one at that.

Canola, which comes from the seed of the edible rape plant, is the most commonly used culinary oil in the world, though the coarse rape green does not have a wide following as a popular vegetable. That's okay, because you'll get the best the plant has to offer by using the oil. Canola oil is a rich source of polyunsaturated fat—it has three times the amount found in olive oil—and it is the lowest among all oils in saturated fat. Its active cancer-fighting qualities come from being one of the richest sources of both omega-3 fatty acids and linoleic acid.

Research shows that canola oil's unique chemistry helps reduce the inflammatory process leading to **prostate cancer**. It can also inhibit progression of the disease in aggressive cases. Another study found that it has an inhibitory effect on **ovarian cancer** cell lines. Omega-3 fatty acids also have been found to be protective against **colon cancer**. Canola oil also has significance for cancer survivors because it has the ability to help slow the growth of residual cancer cells.

If people used canola oil exclusively in place of other vegetable oils, it would provide the necessary daily amount of omega-3s important to health, another study shows.

In the Kitchen with Canola Oil

Canola oil owes its popularity to being so user-friendly. It is sturdy, so it will not wither under high heat like some other oils. Its flavor is mild, making it unobtrusive when you want the natural flavor of foods to come out. It is also much cheaper than olive and boutique oils, such as avocado and walnut oils.

CAULIFLOWER

You'd think that this white-faced crucifer couldn't hold a candle to its deep-green brother, broccoli, but that's not the case at all. Cauliflower's cancer-fighting action comes from its rich content of linolenic acid and polyphenols.

Like broccoli, cauliflower's growth stops at the bud stage, which is why it has such an interesting physique. Some researchers believe this stress enhances its nutritional content.

In the Kitchen with Cauliflower

Cooking, unfortunately, is hard on this vegetable's nutritional content. In one test of 20 popular antioxidant-rich vegetables, cauliflower took the biggest beating. More than 50 percent of its antioxidant content was lost through boiling and microwaving and more than 25 percent was lost during pressure-cooking. To retain its cancer-fighting edge, cook cauliflower gently, if at all. For example:

- Break the heads into little pieces and add them to salads.
- Add florets to vegetable soup during the last five minutes of cooking.
- Use florets in stir-fries. Frying is the method shown to have the least amount of nutritional losses.
- Break off the buds and use them with a dipping sauce as an appetizer.

CARROTS

If you're a smoker, stock up on carrots whenever you're at the supermarket. It just might be your best dietary defense against the ravages of tobacco.

Carrots are a rich source of beta-carotene and retinol, forms of Vitamin A that are well-known defensive weapons against cancer. In one classic study, researchers tested four foods rich in retinol or carotene—carrots, liver, leafy vegetables, and cheese—for their ability to reduce the risk of **lung cancer** in more than 1,200 smokers who had been hospitalized for a tobacco-related ailment. Of the four foods, only carrots and green leafy vegetables proved to be protective. However, of the two, carrots by far offered more protection. Smokers who did not eat carrots had a threefold risk of developing lung cancer over smokers who ate carrots more than once a week. Eating carrots, however, offered no protection against lung cancer in non-smokers and former smokers. This is why researchers believe the nutrients in carrots work synergistically to neutralize the carcinogens in tobacco.

Carrots are not only good for smokers. A four-state survey of the dietary habits of more than 13,000 women found that those who ate the most carrots had a lower risk of **breast cancer** than women who ate the least.

In the Kitchen with Carrots

Fresh, crunchy carrot sticks are one of the best nutritional snacks around, but you'll get even more nutrients from eating them pureed. University of Arkansas researchers measured the antioxidant content of raw and pureed vegetables and found that levels increased by 34 percent the moment they hit the heat. The scientists then stored the carrots for a week and measured again.

The nutrients expanded even more. After that, the nutrient level dropped to that of raw carrots.

There is no reason to be timid about cooking carrots. A major analysis by food scientists in Spain found that the antioxidant activity in carrots *increases* for all cooking methods.

WATER IS A VEGETABLE'S BIGGEST ENEMY

Be careful how you cook vegetables. Some cooking methods can deplete cancer-fighting strength by 50 percent or more. The most egregious? Boiling.

Food scientists in Spain put the 20 top antioxidant-rich vegetables to the most rigorous experiment ever by measuring how their nutrient content survived under the heat of six popular cooking methods—boiling, baking, frying, griddling, microwaving, and pressure cooking. One pound of each vegetable was cooked by each method exactly the same way five different times to assure accuracy.

Boiling, followed by pressure cooking, produced the most loss. Overall, griddling produced the least loss, followed by microwaving and baking. Frying—the testers used olive oil—fell in the middle. Losses ranged anywhere from 5 to more than 50 percent.

CHILI PEPPERS

Chilis, a south-of-the-border staple, are hot, hot, hot in the U.S.A. Lucky for us, because the substance that gives chilis their hot sensation has a long list of health benefits, including the ability to help fight cancer.

Chilis are among the most powerful antioxidants in the plant world, thanks to capsaicin, the substance that gives them their signature heat. Capsaicin is the only thing that sets chilis apart from the many of the world's other peppers. If a pepper has no heat, it has no capsaicin, and if it has no capsaicin, it's not a chili. The more capsaicin, the hotter the chili.

Capsaicin is one mighty powerful healer. In addition to being a potent antioxidant, it also has anti-inflammatory and anti-tumor properties that have been shown to be effective against **leukemia**, **melanoma**, and **prostate cancer**. One study found it to be effective against a type of leukemia that is even resistant to drugs.

Researchers at Cedars-Sinai Medical Center in Los Angeles found that, when taken as a supplement, capsaicin helped promote death in cancerous prostate cells and also helped bring down PSA, a biomarker for the disease, in cancer patients. Used topically, it also can soothe mouth sores in cancer patients undergoing chemotherapy.

In the Kitchen with Chili Peppers

Capsaicin is indestructible. Neither freezing nor cooking can turn down the heat. It is found in the white membrane that holds the seeds—not the seeds themselves, as is commonly believed. If you want to play with fire, select the smallest you can find. Smaller chilis are hotter than large ones.

In order of hotness, the top 10 hottest chilis, and the ones that contain the most capsaicin, are:

1. Red and orange habaneros
2. Scotch Bonnet
3. Thai
4. Red Amazon

5. Pequin
6. Tabasco
7. Serrano
8. Jalapeno
9. New Mexican Red
10. Aji Escabeche

Look for chilis that are firm and have a smooth, glossy outer skin. Generally, the riper, the redder, the hotter. Store fresh peppers in paper towels in the refrigerator, where they will keep for about a week. Or, you can hang them upside down in the sunlight to dry.

With hundreds of different varieties, there is no shortage of culinary adventure. Connoisseurs will tell you that each chili has a distinctive taste and imparts a special flavor to a dish. Here are a few tips for working with chilis:

- Have a separate cutting board and knife just for chilis, if possible. Even washing can't get rid of all the capsaicin.
- Wear plastic food handler gloves when working with chilis and make sure to keep your hands away from your eyes.
- When putting remnants down the garbage disposal, make sure the water is turned on cold. Heat will diffuse the substance in the air—think pepper spray.
- Experiment with chili condiments. Paprika, cayenne, and red pepper flakes are other ways to sprinkle more cancer protection onto your food.

COFFEE

Americans drink a lot of coffee—some 400 million cups are poured in the United States every day. In fact, we drink more coffee per person than any other nation on Earth.

At one time this was a concern among cancer specialists because a handful of studies showed that drinking too much coffee might cause bladder cancer. But not any longer. When the World Cancer Research Fund looked at decades of research it concluded, "Evidence now indicates that coffee is unlikely to have a substantial effect on risk of cancer." Now researchers believe that drinking coffee may actually help *prevent* cancer.

In one study, researchers analyzed more than a dozen studies and found that coffee drinkers had a 41 percent reduced risk of **liver cancer** compared to people who don't drink coffee. Another study of 90,000 Japanese men and women aged 40 to 69 found that those who drank three or more cups of coffee a day had a 50 percent lower risk of **colorectal cancer** than non-coffee drinkers. And scientists in Michigan found that women who drank six or more cups of coffee a day had a 36 percent lower risk of developing non-melanoma **skin cancer**.

So, there's no reason to say *no, thank you* to a cup of coffee. In fact, you should say yes, just for the health of it. Of course, if caffeine keeps you awake, be sure not to have it later in the day.

COLLARD GREENS

This Southern staple and member of the cabbage patch stands out as an anti-cancer food due to its rich content of organosulfur compounds, special phytonutrients that have the ability to trap cancer cells and program their death.

Studies show that organosulfurs contain some 15 different cancer-tracking nutrients that go into action when the leaves are sliced or chewed. Collard greens also are a good source of other important cancer-fighting nutrients, including beta-carotene, calcium vitamins C and E, and zinc. Collards are associated with a reduced risk of **breast**, **esophagus**, **prostate**, **skin** and **ovarian cancers**.

In the Kitchen with Collards

When shopping for collards, pick greens that are rich in color with no sign of yellowing or browning. The smaller the leaves, the more tender the flavor. Refrigerate them, unwashed, in a damp paper towel in a plastic bag. They will keep well for about five days. The best ways to eat them include:

- Steam them for about 30 seconds to 1 minute, or until they just start to turn limp. Drizzle with olive oil heated with garlic.
- Chop and roll them with avocado and cucumber when making sushi rolls.
- Eat them in the traditional Southern style—steamed with black-eyed peas.
- For a different twist, stir-fry collards with tofu, cauliflower florets, and Chinese five-spice powder.

DARK CHOCOLATE

We shouldn't be surprised that dark chocolate has turned out to be such a healthy food. After all, chocolate comes from a plant, just like other health-protecting fruits and vegetables. But chocolate, which comes from the fruit of the cacao tree, is superior to fruits and vegetables in one very special way. It is the richest source of a special class of polyphenols called flavanols, which are well-known cancer fighters.

Eating dark chocolate is a delicious way to protect

yourself against cancer, says Sally Scroggs, a registered dietitian and health education manager at the University of Texas M. D. Anderson Cancer Center in Houston. Recent research shows that the flavanols in dark chocolate play a role in reducing cancer risks by helping to combat cell damage that can lead to tumor growth. These nutrients occur naturally in the cacao bean, the base of all chocolate products.

Cacao beans are, in fact, one of the most concentrated natural sources of antioxidants that exist. Dark chocolate has a higher percentage of healthy antioxidants, without the increased sugar and saturated fats added to milk chocolate, says Scroggs.

Flavonols are concentrated in the cocoa, the solid that is left when cocoa butter is extracted from cacao beans. The higher the flavonol content, the more bitter the taste. "This is the main reason why eating dark chocolate, versus milk or white chocolate, reduces cancer risk," says Scroggs.

In the Candy Shop with Chocolate

Dark chocolate does not have the creamy consistency or sweetness of milk chocolate, but don't let that put you off. Chocolate connoisseurs will argue that cacao content and quality are really what appreciating chocolate is all about.

The American Institute of Cancer Research (AICR) agrees. The more cacao, the better, because as cacao content goes up, sugar comes down. The AICR recommends about an ounce a day for cancer protection.

Here are some tips for getting the most health out of a chocolate indulgence.

- Buy pure dark chocolate containing at least 65 percent cocoa. This is not the kind you buy to make cakes and cookies, which contains more calories, sugar, and unhealthy fats, says Scroggs.

• Buy chocolate in small portions, so you keep portions small. "Remember, dark chocolate is still a calorie-dense food that can be high in fat," says Scroggs. "You can enjoy it daily as part of a balanced diet, as long as you keep your portion size in check."

• Check the ingredients. Make sure the chocolate contains no palm and coconut oils, and it is made without the use of hydrogenated or partially hydrogenated oils.

• Cocoa powder is as nutritious as dark chocolate. Use it for baking and making hot chocolate.

FISH

Where there is seawater there is fish, and where there is fish, there is a lower incidence of cancer. It's a fact that has researchers debating: Is eating fish so healthy that it can reduce the risk of cancer? Or, is the risk of cancer lower among fish eaters because they consume less red meat?

Though it could take years for scientists to solve this conundrum, there is no reason it should get in the way of your menu planning, because there is enough evidence to show that a few servings of fish a week belongs on an anti-cancer diet.

One of the first observations that fueled this debate was a study reported in the *British Journal of Cancer* almost a decade ago that compared the rate of **lung cancer** between Japanese and Americans. Lung cancer is the leading cause of cancer death in both nations, but the Japanese cancer rate is less than two-thirds the U.S. rate. Researchers have long speculated this is largely due to the difference in diet between the two. The Japanese eat a healthier diet that relies on fish, soy, and green tea, compared to Americans, who have a diet higher in saturated fat. The study, which compared the dietary and lifestyle habits of more than 4,000 Japanese men, postulated that eating large amounts of fish high in omega-3 fatty acids was helping to protect them from lung cancer. The researchers also found that people who ate the most cooked or raw fish had a lung cancer risk nearly half that of people who ate the least amount of fish. They didn't find the same effect, however, among people who ate dried or salted fish. This bolstered the argument even more, because the production process destroys the fatty acids in fish.

A few years later, another British medical journal, *The Lancet*, reported a study conducted in Sweden, where there is also a high consumption of fatty fish. After analyzing the diets of 2,600 men, researchers found that eating just one serving of salmon a week reduced the risk of developing **prostate cancer** by 43 percent. Again the credit went to salmon's high omega-3 content.

Most of the research on cancer and fish consumption, however, has concentrated on **colorectal cancer**. Numerous studies have found that eating red meat is associated with an increased risk, but trials trying to associate eating fish with reduced risk have been inconsistent. Recent major studies in Europe and the United States, however, indicate that eating fish plays an important role in preventing colorectal cancer. In the European study, Polish researchers spent five years following the dietary habits of patients admitted to the hospital as a result of precancerous or cancerous polyps. They found that risk increased with meat consumption and "was significantly reduced" with moderate fish intake, defined as one to two servings a week.

The major U.S. Physicians Health Study compared the dietary intake of red meat and fish over the course of 22 years and found that those who ate the most fish (an average of 26.1 times a month) had a lower risk of colorectal cancer than those who ate the least (an average of 2.2 times a month).

The bottom line: Eat fish as a substitute for red meat as much as possible, but a minimum of once or twice a week.

Mercury Is Going Up

There is another conundrum to this fish tale and it involves worldwide concern over the increasing amount of mercury in fish. All fish contains mercury, but it is highest in fatty fish, such as tuna and salmon, which also happen to be the most popular kinds of fish eaten in the United States. A 2009 study reported in *Environmental Health Perspectives* found that many U.S. women have mercury blood levels above what is generally considered safe. Asians, Hawaiians, and high-income women living in the Northeast are at high risk. Women in New York City are at the highest risk.

All finfish and shellfish contain mercury, according to the U.S. Environmental Protection Agency (EPA). Though most doctors and the EPA feel that the benefits of eating fish outweigh the risks, they say that women of childbearing age should eat fish cautiously. Mercury poisoning has a long list of side effects, but it carries the greatest risk to a fetus. To get benefit without risk, the EPA recommends these guidelines for pregnant women and women considering getting pregnant:

- Do not eat shark, swordfish, king mackerel, or tilefish. Larger fatty fish attract more mercury than smaller fish.

- Eat a variety of other fish, including shrimp, halibut, and trout. In the study, women with the highest blood levels of mercury ate mostly salmon or tuna. Limit fish consumption to two average servings a week. An average serving is considered 6 ounces.
- Limit your intake of white albacore canned tuna to 6 ounces per week, as it contains more mercury than light tuna.

Here are some other ways to ensure they you are eating fish with the least amounts of mercury.

Choose wild salmon over farm raised. Americans, by far, are the biggest salmon eaters. According to the Institute for Health and the Environment, Americans eat 207,000 metric tons of salmon a year. This popularity has increased the number of commercial fish farms—and also has raised another health concern. Studies have found that farmed salmon contains more environmental toxins that those caught in the sea, because the close breeding grounds are more attractive to contaminants.

Ask the right questions. Supermarkets are the most popular outlets for farm-raised salmon and, reportedly, some markets try to pass off farm-raised fish as wild. If the fish is not marked "wild," specifically ask the fishmonger if the fish you are buying was farm-raised.

If you're still not so sure, ask where the salmon was fished. If it's from Chile, it is most likely farmed. Chile is the world's second-largest producer of farm-raised salmon, and most of the salmon sold in the United States comes from Chile or Canada. A tipoff that you may not be getting wild salmon is price. Wild salmon is far more expensive than farm-raised and can cost from $15 to $20 a pound.

In the end, you'll know if you're eating wild salmon by the taste. Buttery-textured wild salmon is fins and tails superior to farm-raised. Wild salmon also contains more omega-3s than farm-raised.

In the Kitchen with Fish

Women may make the greatest effort to eat the most fish, but the typical American isn't eating enough to get a cancer-protecting effect. According to statistics, the average American eats fish about once every ten days. If you're one of them, all you need to do is eat two more servings a month to get the minimum cancer-protective effect. You'd be best off making your choices from the fish with the highest levels of omega-3s. They are, in order of content:

- Herring
- Sardines
- Salmon
- Mackerel
- Trout
- Halibut
- Tuna

Here are some tips to get the most out of your fish meals at home:

- The most convenient way to boost your fish intake is to eat tuna salads or sandwiches made with canned tuna. White albacore is the most popular, but it contains more mercury than light tuna and is also more expensive. Whichever you eat, get fish packed in water instead of oil. It will keep down calories and fat.

- Eat fish steamed, poached or baked. Frying reduces omega-3 levels and also causes the build up of heterocyclic amines (HCAs), known carcinogens. (For more information on HCAs, see Marinades on page 111.)
- Here is an easy and delicious way to enjoy salmon or other fish with a similar texture, such as sea bass. Place a thick fish fillet on a large piece of aluminum foil set on a baking sheet. Dice onions and tomato and mix with a tablespoon or two of olive oil and a pinch of oregano and marjoram. Cover the salmon with the mixture, sprinkle with chives, and fold the ends of the foil up tent-like. Seal tightly. Bake at 350°F for 30 minutes or until it reaches desired doneness.

GARLIC

Garlic, the most powerfully flavored member of the odiferous onion family, is an indispensable ingredient in many cuisines. And it is no coincidence that these cuisines—most notably those in India, Asia and the Mediterranean basin—are also among the healthiest in the world.

Garlic has a unique and complex chemistry that creates a chain of bioactivity when you smash a garlic clove on a cutting board with the flat edge of a knife. Most distinct is the release of allicin, an organosulfur compound responsible for the bulb's moniker "the stinking herb." This highly reactive compound is also why garlic is considered a super food credited with helping boost immunity and protecting against a host of health threats, including cancer.

Nearly 100 animal and human studies have linked

consumption of raw or cooked garlic to fighting a variety of cancers. Five out of eight human studies and 11 animal studies show that daily consumption of culinary garlic can reduce the incidence of **colorectal cancer** by 30 percent. Numerous studies have found it to be protective against **prostate cancer**.

In China, where the rate of **stomach cancer** is high, researchers found that those who consumed a half-ounce of garlic a day had a tenfold reduced risk of dying from the disease than those who ate less than one clove.

Scientists are not certain how garlic fights cancer, but suspect that different bioactive responses work in tandem to suppress proliferation of cancer cells and cause their death. One Chinese study, for example, found that garlic has the ability to annihilate *H. pylori,* bacteria that eventually can lead to stomach cancer. Another study conducted in Jordan found that dietary garlic, when combined with soy food such as tofu, can help protect mammary glands from the oxidative stress that causes **breast cancer**. Studies show it has the potential to neutralize toxins that cause **bladder cancer**.

Garlic cooked or eaten raw also has been associated with a reduced risk of **leukemia** and **cervix, esophagus, larynx, lung, kidney, oral**, and **ovarian cancers**.

In the Kitchen with Garlic

Allicin has strong working action, just as its odor suggests, and can withstand just about any cooking method.

Here are a few ways to get more garlic in your diet:

- Dice it, slice it, smash it, or mince it. It doesn't matter, as long as you can smell it.

• If you think your stomach can't hold up to eating whole garlic cloves, you have not tried roasted garlic. It's easy to make, too. Just take an entire head of garlic and remove all the loose skin. Most of the skin should remain intact. Place the head in a piece of tinfoil. Fold up the sides, sprinkle a tablespoon of olive oil on top, wrap it tightly, and roast in a pan or on a cookie sheet at 375°F until soft.

• Scatter peeled garlic cloves among root vegetables when roasting.

GREEN TEA

Sit, relax, sip a cup of green tea, and enjoy the moment.

Yes, just the thought of a warm cup of tea sounds soothing, and it should be even more comforting to know that with every cup comes a serving of good health. No wonder the beverage has been a leading favorite the world over for centuries!

Green tea is loaded with catechins, special substances with known anti-cancer activity, but its real strength comes from a special brand of catchins called epigallocatechin gallate (EGCG). EGCG is a particularly potent, cell-protecting antioxidant with many proven health benefits, including the ability to help prevent at least 10 types of cancer.

No nation drinks more tea than China, where 10 cups a day is considered normal. So, it's no surprise that virtually all the studies on green tea and health have been conducted in China.

When it comes to cancer, EGCG has a take-no-prisoners attitude. It can go after cancer cells like an assassin, tailing them and taking them out when they refuse to die. It spies on genes, too, and has the ability to smother them before they commit cell mutiny. It can turn into a double agent and masquerade as a free radical inside a tumor cell, then turn on it like a suicide bomber. It also does duty as an EMT in the liver, where it helps pump new life into cells assaulted by toxins.

In 2008, Chinese experts did a meta-analysis of hundreds of studies spanning more than 40 years to ascertain green tea's true strength as a cancer fighter. They found that 58 percent of the studies supported an association between long-term tea consumption and a reduced cancer risk. They found the greatest protection comes from drinking five or more cups a day, but even drinking one cup offers some defense.

The Drink for Hard Livers

Green tea is somewhat of a patron saint for drinkers and smokers. In one study, green tea reduced the rate of **liver cancer** by a remarkable 78 percent in alcoholics and 43 percent in smokers.

Consider the soothing feeling as tea goes down the throat and it's no surprise that the strongest evidence on the protective power of green tea was found for cancers of the gastrointestinal tract. The Chinese analysis found that green tea offers a significant reduction in the risk of **esophageal** and **oral cancers** among women (though not men). There is a strong association between tea consumption and reduced risk of **colorectal cancer** in both men and women. Results, however, were mixed for **stomach** and **breast cancers**.

Green tea helps protect men against **prostate cancer** and it reduces the risk of **endometrial cancer** in women prior to menopause. It also improves the survival rate for **ovarian cancer**. Several studies have found a protective effect against **pancreatic cancer** and one study found it reduces the risk of **leukemia.** Mayo Clinic researchers report positive results from early studies using EGCG to treat patients with leukemia.

In the Kitchen with Green Tea

Because tea generally does not spoil, it can be stored and will last forever. Unfortunately, catechins do not, according to research conducted jointly in Korea and California. They stored green tea under prime conditions (a cool, dark place) and tested for catechin loss every week. At the start of the sixth month, they noticed catechin had degraded 28 percent. A month later the loss was 50 percent.

So, buy tea according to your drinking habits. Since you most likely won't know how long the tea has been sitting on a store's shelf, buy enough to last no more than a month or two.

To get the most protection out of green, drink *at least* five cups a day. That's a lot of tea, if you aren't a regular tea or coffee drinker, but if you sip it as you do water—and instead of diet soda!—you can easily reach five cups a day. Here are a few tips on how to enhance the tea drinking experience:

- Drink it iced, just as you would black tea. As it steeps, add some mint leaves, which also possess anti-cancer activity.
- Make a chai by brewing it in milk and adding cinnamon and nutmeg.
- Freeze it in ice cube trays, then crush the cubes in a blender to make a slush.
- Blend it with tropical fruits, such as papaya and mango, with low-fat milk and a drop of vanilla, to make a smoothie.

CAUTION: Several studies found that drinking liquids that are too hot, particularly tea, increases the risk of **esophageal cancer**. In Iran, where the incidence of esophageal cancer is high, people love hot tea and drink an average of 33 ounces a day. And it appears they are paying an unfair price. Hot tea is the source of their high cancer rate, according to a study of 48,582 Iranians. Risk was considerably greater among those who drank tea at a temperature of 149°F or greater than for those who drank it lukewarm or at room temperature. Wait four minutes or longer after tea steeps before drinking it, suggest the researchers.

KALE

Like other cruciferous vegetables, this curly green on a cabbage-like stem is brimming with the same cancer-fighting nutrients as the rest of its family. What makes kale stand out, however, is our ability to better absorb its calcium, an important mineral that helps fight **colorectal cancer**.

In the first ever study to examine absorbency in calcium-rich foods, kale came in Numero Uno. It came in head-to-head with milk (which is only fortified with calcium), and left spinach in the dust. Leaf for leaf, kale contains three times as much calcium as spinach, which until this study got all the accolades for being a super source of calcium.

Why Kale's So Cool

When you take a whiff of kale, you get a heady scent of sulphur. This comes from sulforaphane, the same lung-protecting substance that makes broccoli an anti-cancer superstar. Kale is also rich in flavonoids, like other crucifers, and contains 32 other health-rendering compounds. Together they have the ability to bind bile acids and help prevent tumor formation.

Kale should be on the menu of those at risk for bladder cancer. In one study of nearly 1,500 people, University of Texas researchers found that people with the lowest intake of cruciferous vegetables, such as kale, had the highest risk for **bladder cancer**.

Kale is an excellent course of vitamin C, a vitamin with cancer-fighting strength. Just one cup of cooked kale supplies almost the full daily value.

In the Kitchen with Kale

When shopping for kale, look for a firm stem with deeply colored leaves. Select heads with smaller leaves, as they will be more tender and mild. Refrigerate, unwashed, in a damp paper towel in a sealed bag to keep it from wilting. Kale leaves tend to be dirty, so make sure to wash them well before using.

Kale is rather coarse and strongly flavored, which does not make it as popular as other leafy greens. However, it has the versatility of spinach and can be made in a variety of tasty ways. Here are a few ideas.

- Steam it until the leaves are barely limp. This is a terrific cooking method because steaming increases bile-binding activity. Sprinkle with your favorite herbs.
- Try kale with pasta. Make a sauce by sautéing shallots and garlic in olive oil. Add a quarter cup each of white wine and chicken broth and bring to a simmer. Turn off the heat, add the kale, and let it wilt. Turn in cooked pasta. Serve with feta cheese sprinkled on top.
- Kale pairs well with apple. Steam the kale slightly, then squeeze out any accumulated water. Heat

olive oil in a sauté pan and add garlic and chopped apples. Add the kale and stir until heated through. Throw in broken walnut pieces and sprinkle with red wine vinegar just before serving.

LEMONS AND LIMES

Do lemons and limes conjure up images of sunshine and warmth? Or maybe they remind you of a child-hood lemonade stand or a tall tropical drink garnished with umbrella-speared fruit.

Lemons and limes are the quintessential sunshine fruit. There is possibly no food, and certainly no fruit, as ubiquitous as these citrus pals. Lemons and limes need the brilliant warmth of year-round sunshine to grow, which is likely why researchers pondered if they held any secret beneath their skin. Could these sun-kissed fruits protect human skin from the ravages of the sun?

Researchers tested this theory on a group of older residents with no signs of skin cancer, despite decades of living in the Sun Belt region of southern Arizona, which also happens to be the skin cancer capital of the United States. Sure enough, they turned out to be citrus lovers. More than 65 percent reported eating citrus fruit weekly, mostly oranges and grapefruit, and even more drank the fruits' juice. The researchers could not, however, find a connection between their love of citrus fruit and reduced rate of skin cancer. That is, until they picked up on an important detail. They noticed that 35 percent had reported that they routinely ate the *peel* of lemons and limes (known as the zest) in their cooking and drinks. They found the connection!

"Not only is peel consumption common," noted the

researchers, "there was a dose-response relationship between citrus peel consumption and human cancers."

Citrus fruit has a number of health benefits, thanks to limonene, the active ingredient abundant in citrus fruit. And, no surprise, limonene is concentrated in the peel.

In addition to **skin cancer**, studies have found that limonene helps fight **breast**, **colon**, **lung**, **oral** and **stomach cancers**. The Arizona finding, though preliminary, found that the limonene in lemons and limes helps prevent damaged cells under the skin from proliferating.

In the Kitchen with Lemons and Limes
For all their nose-puckering tartness, lemons and limes are surprisingly refreshing. Lemon and lime zest is commonly used in flavoring desserts and drinks, so consider this when buying. Organic fruits are your best bet, but whatever you buy, make sure to wash them well before using. Look for fruit with blemish-free skin and brilliant color. They can be kept at room temperature for about a week, as long as you keep them out of the sun. They will stay fresh a while longer if you refrigerate them as soon as you buy them.

To extract the most juice from a lemon or lime, roll it first along a hard surface. You can cut the peel by using a zester or paring knife.

Lemons and limes go with just about everything, so use them at will. Here are a few ideas:

- For any recipes that call for lemon or lime juice, add a teaspoon of chopped zest.
- Put lemon or lime peel under the skin of chicken before baking.
- Cut up a lemon or two and put it inside the cavity of a whole chicken when roasting.

- Place sliced lemons and limes under whole fish or on top of fish fillets when baking.
- Add zest to meat and vegetable stews.

MANGO

The mango is the quintessential exotic fruit. Its soft and succulent flesh clings to a large, rock-solid pit that is impossible to remove, which leaves many wondering: *What the heck are you supposed to do with a mango?!* Well, it's time to learn, because the mango just may turn out to be one of the most important fruits in the anti-cancer arsenal.

As its brilliant orange flesh suggests, the mango is rich in antioxidants, including beta carotene, vitamins A and C, and quercitin. Mangoes, however, possess an antioxidant makeup in both variety and quantity that makes them unique in the fruit world—and cancer prevention.

Mango is native to India, where it is revered as "the king of all fruit," so it's no surprise that it is also the land of mango research. Indian scientists are focused on a key nutrient called lupeol, which they believe may be able to reduce the incidence of **prostate cancer**. In one recent experiment, scientists injected male mice with enough testosterone to make the prostate grow. For the next two weeks, half the mice received supplemental lupeol in their mouse chow; the other half got no lupeol. Meanwhile, they watched to see what happened. They saw prostates grow in the lupeol-deprived mice, but not in the lupeol-fed mice.

In another lab experiment, the same researchers tested the effects of lupeol on human cancer cells and found it helped alter DNA activity that leads to tumor formation.

Earlier lab studies at the University of Florida found

that mango juice inhibited the growth cycle of cells leading to both **prostate** and **pancreatic cancer**. In other experiments, lupeol impaired tumor growth of hard-to-treat head and neck cancers, including **esophageal**, **laryngeal**, **oral cavity**, **pharyngeal**, and **salivary gland cancers**. It also had the same effect on less-threatening **thyroid cancer**.

"We think mangoes have some unique antioxidants as well as quantities of antioxidants that might not be found in other fruits and vegetables," commented the Florida researchers.

In the Kitchen with Mangoes

You could say that no two mangoes look alike. They can be many shades of red, green, or yellow, or a variety of all three colors. But don't worry about color when trying to select a good one, as it has nothing to do with freshness. You want to choose a mango based on its firmness and when you plan to eat it.

Mangoes are ripened off the tree, which makes them great for export. When ripe, a mango will give with a gentle squeeze. If you are not planning on using it right away, find one that is firmer to the touch. Also, sniff the ends of the fruit. A ripe mango will give off a mellow aroma.

Unripe mangos should be kept at room temperature. To speed up the ripening process, put them in a brown paper bag. Once ripe, put them in the refrigerator.

Mangoes are quite easy to handle, once you know how to do it. The secret to handling the pit is to *not* handle it at all. Here's what to do:

• Wash the mango and place it on a cutting board on its side, not on the stem end.

- Take a sharp knife and position it about an inch from center and slice clear through. Do the same to the other side. You now have two cheeks.
- To make fruit slices, hold a cheek in the palm of one hand and slice lengthwise, but not through the skin. Hold each end with your thumb and index figure and turn the fruit inside out. Sever the fruit from the skin.
- To dice the fruit, slice the flesh crosswise. Turn the cheek inside out and cut the fruit from the skin.
- Toss the center core with the pit in the trash. Do not attempt to put it down the garbage disposal.

Mango most commonly is eaten out of hand. It is also popular in chutneys and salsa. It pairs tastefully with diced tomatoes, green peppers, onions and a little chopped cilantro to make a fast and easy salsa. Grill slices and serve atop barbecued chicken breasts.

MARINADES

There is nothing like the mention of grilling and cancer to spoil a good barbecue. But not at your house! You're about to discover the secret to safe grilling, and it's a tasty one, too. In one word, it's *marinate*.

Researchers at Kansas State University have found that marinating can prevent carcinogenic compounds from forming in meat, poultry, and fish that is grilled, fried or broiled at high temperature.

Studies show that cooking these foods at temperatures above 352°F for more than four minutes produces compounds called heterocyclic amines (HCAs). Another class of carcinogens, called polycyclic aromatic hydrocarbons (PAHs), form when smoke and flame-ups from fat drippings cause food to char. Both are associated with **breast**, **colon**, **pancreatic** and **stomach cancers.**

The researchers found that you can deflect this cancer risk simply by marinating food before grilling. In their experiment, they immersed round steak in one of three commercial spice-containing marinades—Caribbean, southwest and herb—for one hour, then grilled it at 400°F. The Caribbean blend had the highest resistance to HCAs, showing an 88 percent decrease. The herb blend reduced formation of HCAs by 72 percent, and the southwest blend by 57 percent. The researchers believe the antioxidants in herbs and other common marinade ingredients helped resist HCA formation.

You can make your own marinades by using any of these antioxidant-rich herbs and condiments in a combination with liquids, such as oil, water, soy sauce and vinegar:

- Basil
- Cayenne pepper
- Chili sauce
- Citrus juice—lemon, lime, orange
- Garlic
- Marjoram
- Mint
- Mustard seeds
- Onion
- Oregano
- Peppercorns
- Rosemary
- Sage
- Savory
- Tabasco
- Thyme

Make grilling extra-safe by following these guidelines.

- Avoid charring food by turning it frequently. Scrape any charred flesh off before serving.
- Reduce fatty flare-ups by trimming meats and removing skin from poultry.
- Serve red meats medium rare. HCAs build with length of cooking.
- Put meat or poultry in the microwave for a minute or two before grilling to reduce the length of time on the grill.
- Choose lean cuts of meat, instead of high-fat varieties such as ribs or sausages.
- Avoid piercing with a fork, which allows juices to escape and cause flame-ups.
- Keep meat portions small to reduce grilling time. Skewered kebabs cook the fastest.

MUSTARD SEED

If you think the best you'll get out of biting into a ballpark frank is great taste, then you're in for a bonus—as long as you smear your frank with mustard.

Mustard is made from the seeds of mustard greens, which get their healing qualities from fine breeding—they come from the cancer-fighting cruciferous clan. Though mustard greens contain the same cancer-fighting compounds found in kale and cabbage, it is the ferulic acid found in the seeds that makes this spice a potent cancer fighter. (Mustard seeds actually come from any of three non-edible mustard greens.)

Though mighty small, there is a lot of might in a tablespoon of mustard seeds. The seeds are a concentrated source of multiple compounds with anti-cancer activity that enhances the immune system's antioxidant defense system. "Their inclusion in the diet may very probably contribute to reducing the risk of cancer incidence in the human population," reported the *Comprehensive Reviews in Food Science and Food Safety* in 2009.

In the Kitchen with Mustard

To keep their flavor fresh, do not refrigerate mustards. Instead, keep bottles of homemade yellow and brown mustards on a condiment tray.

Mustards come in an infinite number of flavors, strengths, and colors, and chefs around the world take great pride in their national brand. Dijon may be their most popular mustard, but the French actually have hundreds of different varieties to boast about. England and Germany are also well-known for their unique mustards.

Mustard seeds are usually fried to impart their flavor. Mustard powder itself does not have much taste, but once you mix it with cold water, enzymes go into action that bring out pungency and heat. Prepared mustard, mustard powder, and mustard seeds can be used in your culinary adventures. Here are some ideas:

- Mustard goes well with lamb and chicken. Just coat the flesh well with prepared mustard, sprinkle on herbs of your choice, and bake.
- Add mustard seeds to marinades.
- Mustard is the secret to a true French vinaigrette. Put a small dollop of mustard in a shallow bowl, and whisk while adding a stream of olive oil and balsamic or red wine vinegar (a ratio of four parts

oil to one part vinegar). Add garlic, if desired, and your favorite herbs.

- Add prepared mustard to potato salad and powdered mustard to chicken salad.
- Do as the Germans do, and use dark, grainy mustard as a condiment on boiled potatoes or beef.
- Mix prepared mustard with honey, soy sauce, and Asian spices, such as five-spice powder, to make a dipping sauce for dumplings.
- Substitute prepared mustard for high-fat mayonnaise for sandwiches and team it with onions instead of ho-hum ketchup on burgers.

OLIVE OIL

Olive oil is perfect proof that it isn't fat, but the type of fat, that is important when it comes to good health and longevity. Just look at the Mediterranean diet. Though it is low in meat and abundant in locally grown fresh fruit, vegetables, and fish, it is also high in fat—fat that comes almost exclusively from olive oil.

People who live in Greece and other areas along the Mediterranean love olive oil and use it in abundance. Scientists from around the world have been studying the lifestyle of the Greeks for years and believe that their locally grown diet in general and olive oil in particular is the reason they enjoy the lowest incidence in the world for many types of cancers.

Olive oil plays a unique role in cancer prevention. Scientists believe many of the same characteristics in olive oil that are so well-known for protecting the heart are also helping to protect us from cancer.

Olive oil is the highest source of monounsaturated fat, the so-called health-promoting "good fat." Monos are special because they contain oleic acid, a compound researchers believe have the potential to target and deactivate the genes linked to **breast** and **ovarian cancers**. For example, when researchers from Northwestern University in Chicago exposed two strains of genetically acquired aggressive **breast cancer** to oleic acid, resistance to the disease increased by 46 percent. In another study, oleic acid increased the effectiveness of a drug used to treat the cancer. And that's just the beginning.

Numerous studies are proving that olive oil's true anti-cancer armor comes from its unique profile of powerful polyphenols that fight cancer in a variety of other ways. This special makeup is found only in the finest of olive oils, those labeled *extra virgin*. Extra virgin olive oil contains 30 different polyphenols, each with their own demonstrated anti-cancer qualities. The most important are squalene, lignans, and tyrosol, nutrients associated with a reduced risk of **breast**, **colon**, **prostate**, **skin**, **stomach** and **upper respiratory tract cancers**.

What It Takes to Be Extra Virgin

Walk into any grocery shop or home in Greece, and you will find only the finest olive oil, made by small, family-run operations using old-fashioned manufacturing customs. These are known to be the best olive oils in the world—cloudy, slightly thick, and deep golden green, the sign that the oil is extra virgin.

To be extra virgin, the oil must be painstakingly extracted from the fruit without altering the oil and without any treatment other than washing, decanting and filtration.

Extra-virgin oil is particularly beneficial to gastrointestinal health. When researchers simulated the human digestive system, only extra-virgin oil had the strength to ameliorate *H. pylori*, a stubborn and resistant bacterium that causes chronic inflammation that can lead to **stomach cancer**.

OLIVES ARE GOOD FOR YOU, TOO

Olives possess the same anti-cancer characteristics as olive oil, but don't expect to reap these healthy benefits from eating the kind of olives found in a martini.

The healthiest olives are the fruity-flavored ripe black olives from Greece, Italy, and France. They feel and taste oily, compared to the brined green Spanish olives that go in a cocktail.

If you want to add a pinch of health to your martini, you're better off substituting an onion (see Onions on page 120) and calling your drink a Gibson.

In the Kitchen with Olive Oil

It doesn't take therapeutic doses of olive oil to achieve cancer-protecting benefits. Many studies have found that ordinary, everyday culinary use of olive oil in place of butter will strengthen your cancer armor exponentially. For example, one study of 3,442 women in Italy who cooked exclusively with olive oil found they had a lower risk of **ovarian cancer** than women who used butter and olive oil.

The best olive oils come from the first pressing and

range from golden yellow to almost bright green in color. The quality of olive oil is dependent on its acid content—the more refining, or filtering, it goes through, the higher the acid level. The greener the oil, the less acid it contains. Extra-virgin olive oil is deep gold to brilliant green in color. To be labeled *extra virgin*, the acid content cannot be more than 1 percent. Look for the designation *extra nonfiltre* on the label.

Olive oil is somewhat temperamental. Not only can it turn rancid quite easily, it can also lose its nutritive value if it sits around too long. One Italian study figured out the nutritional shelf life of olive oil by allowing it to sit in storage under normal conditions for six months and testing its nutritive value every few weeks. The oil was fine up to three months, then polyphenol content started to break down. By six months, the cancer-protecting nutrients had diminished 40 percent.

Extra-virgin olive oil is expensive (but worth it), so you want to make sure to handle it carefully. Here's what to do:

- Buy no more than the amount you figure you'll use in one to two months' time. Although antioxidants remain intact for three months, consider that your purchase has also been on the shelf for an unknown amount of time.
- The delicate chemical composition of olive oil deteriorates in light and heat, so keep it in an opaque bottle and in a cool, dark place. The ideal temperature is between 68° and 77°F.
- Store olive oil in small containers. The headspace in the bottle collects oxygen, which causes oxidation. Use a bottle no larger than 1 liter, about 4 cups.
- Extra-virgin olive oil has a low smoking point

(250°F), so keep the heat low in the frying pan. If your recipe calls for very high heat, use canola oil.

MAKING A BIG FAT CHANGE

The Mediterranean diet may be high in fat, but it is low in saturated fat—and that makes a big fat difference. Butter is almost all saturated fat.

The two most important dietary changes you can make to reduce your odds of getting cancer are to eat lots of fruit and vegetables every day and reduce your intake of saturated fat. More and more studies are pointing to saturated fat as a real troublemaker, especially when it comes to **breast**, **colorectal**, and **stomach cancers**.

You can take a big step in reducing fat intake in your diet by eliminating butter from your life. Substitute butter for one of these nutritious oils, which contain less than 2 grams of saturated fat per tablespoon.

Oil	Gram per tablespoon
Canola	1.0
Almond	1.1
Safflower	1.2
Sunflower	1.4
Avocado	1.6
Olive	1.9

The best way to appreciate the full-bodied flavor of olive oil is in its natural state, such as a dressing for salads, but there are plenty of ways to be creative. Here are a few suggestions:

- Put olive oil in a small, pretty, dark-colored bottle and keep it on the table in place of butter. Keep a bottle of mixed Italian herbs next to it, so it's easy to mix an herb dipping sauce for bread instead of serving bread and butter at mealtime.
- Add olive oil and pureed roasted garlic to mashed potatoes.
- Drizzle olive oil on steamed or grilled vegetables.
- Make "fried" chicken by coating it with fresh bread-crumbs mixed into olive oil and bake at 425°F until golden.
- Put olive oil in a small spray bottle to oil baking pans.
- Spray French fries with olive oil and bake in the oven at 450°F until crisp.

ONIONS

Lewis and Clark, Amos and Andy, Jack and Jill, Garlic and Onions. For some famous duos, it's hard to mention one without the other.

Garlic and onions reign over a kingdom of vegetables called the *Allium* family, a large clan that includes chives, leeks, shallots, scallions, and dozens of other variations of these outstanding culinary bulbs. They emit a special friendly weapon named allicin that makes its presence known whenever they enter anyone's air space. Though each brings its own brand of chemistry to the tumor-fighting front, onions are an Allium of unique distinction.

As a stand-alone, onions' reputation is well documented—and not only because they are the only vegetable that can make a person cry. Onions possess more phytochemicals than any member of the Allium clan and are the third richest source of cancer-fighting flavonols (next to broccoli and spinach) among all vegetables. Onions are also one of the few foods containing hydoxybenzoic acid, a special type of phytonutrient that makes antioxidants fight even harder. Plus, they are a rare source of quercitin, which has cancer-fighting power of its own.

Onions get their signature tear-jerk reaction from allyl sulfate, a sulphur-smelling phytonutrient in allicin that is released when a knife slashes through the onion's membranes. The stronger the onion, the stronger the sulphur, the stronger the nutrient content.

All this special goodness gives onions a powerful ability to help fight cancer. Onions have proven to be even more powerful than garlic against several types of cancer. When researchers compared the biggest onion eaters to the biggest garlic eaters, they found that:

- Garlic reduced the risk of **esophageal cancer** by 57 percent, but onions reduced it by 88 percent.
- Garlic reduced the risk of **pharyngeal cancer** by 39 percent, but onions reduced it 84 percent.
- Garlic reduced the risk of **laryngeal cancer** by 44 percent, but onions reduced it by 83 percent.
- Garlic reduced the risk of **ovarian cancer** by 22 percent, but onions reduced it by 73 percent.
- Garlic reduced the risk of **prostate cancer** by 19 percent, but onions reduced it by 71 percent.
- Garlic reduced the risk of **kidney cancer** by 31 percent, but onions reduced it by 38 percent.
- Garlic reduced the risk of **breast cancer** by 10 percent, but onions reduced it by 25 percent.

Together, however, garlic and onions make a powerful team. Together they have been found to resist **leukemia**, **brain**, **endometrial**, **lung** and **stomach cancers**.

For example, a study in the Netherlands showed that people who ate two to three helpings of onions a week had a moderately lower risk of stomach cancer than people who ate a few servings a week. A study in China, however, found that people who ate onions *and* garlic daily had a tenfold greater reduction in stomach cancer risk than those who didn't.

One Hawaiian study of onions alone found an association with a reduced risk of lung cancer. Another study found it helped protect against squamous cell carcinoma, a type of non-melanoma skin cancer. In both studies, the anti-cancer effect was attributed to the high content of quercitin in onions.

In the Kitchen with Onions

You can help guard against cancer by eating as little as one to two servings of onions a week, but eating onions daily is best. Of all the many varieties, yellow onions are the strongest and, therefore, have the most anti-cancer activities. Vidalia onions, the sweet and mildest variety, contain the least. Delicate shallots pack a lot of power for their size. Ounce for ounce, they have six times as many flavonols as Vidalia onions and have even more antioxidant activity than the robust yellow onion.

Buy onions that are firm and uniform in color, without any dark blemishes. They are best stored at room temperature away from sunlight. Stronger onions are hardier and will keep in a cool place for at least two months without spoiling. And there is no need to be cautious about how you cook them, because their nutrient content stands up to any type of cooking, except boiling. In fact, griddling and microwaving increases some of their antioxidant activity.

Here are some other tips to make handling onions easier.

- Cut back on a tearful production when working with onions by refrigerating them beforehand. The cold slows the volatility of allicin but does not destroy it.
- Do not cut an onion under running water. It washes away the allicin and sends its cancer-fighting power down the drain.
- Don't store onions with potatoes. They will absorb moisture from potatoes and both will turn rancid.
- You can chop onions in advance and store them tightly wrapped in the refrigerator for up to two days.

ORANGES AND TANGERINES

A toxic lifestyle is hard on the body, particularly the organ mainly responsible for taking in oxygen—the esophagus. Several years ago researchers in Shanghai wanted to find out if high consumption of fruit, seafood, and milk—the area's dietary staples—offered smokers and drinkers any protection against **esophageal cancer**.

They recruited 18,244 middle-aged and older men at risk for esophageal cancer and divided them into two groups. The high-risk group included long-term heavy smokers or drinkers. The low-risk group included less habitual users of tobacco and alcohol. After adjusting for all risk factors, they determined that the heavy drinkers and smokers had a twofold increased risk of developing esophageal cancer over the less-habitual group. With that established, they set out to follow their dietary habits and tested them for cancer signs for the next several years.

The researchers found that heavy smokers and drinkers who had the highest intake of fruit had a 40 to

60 percent reduced cancer risk compared to those with the lowest intake. The foods that they ate the most? Oranges and tangerines.

Oranges and tangerines are a super source of anti-oxidant vitamin C, which helps protect against infection with *H. pylori*, the bacterium that causes ulcers and, in turn, can cause **stomach cancer**. One long-term national study called the Third National Health and Nutrition Examination Survey found that people with the highest levels of vitamin C had the lowest incidence of infection from *H. pylori*. If you've had problems with *H. pylori,* make an orange or orange juice part of your daily diet.

In the Kitchen with Oranges

To get the most nutrition out of oranges, eat them when they are fully ripe and almost at the point of turning rancid. Austrian researchers found that this is the peak of their antioxidant activity.

Choose oranges and tangerines that are large and firm with a smoothly textured skin. Smaller oranges generally are juicier than large oranges. Both fruits can be kept at room temperature or stored in the refrigerator. Either way, they will last for several weeks.

Make sure to wash them well before eating them. Pesticides, dirt, and grit can accumulate on their skin.

Tangerines are generally eaten out of hand but oranges are extremely versatile and go with just about anything. They can play a main or supporting role in everything from appetizer to dessert. They are also the source of the most popular beverage—orange juice. Here are a few ideas for getting more versatility out of oranges.

- If you are going to juice oranges, make sure they are at room temperature. This ensures you will get the maximum juice from the fruit. Roll each one on the counter a few times to help release the juice.

- Pair them with greens in salads.
- Cut them into pieces and throw on top of ice cream.
- Peel and section an orange and freeze them on a baking sheet. Then put them in a freeze-lock bag. Use them like ice cubes in summer tonics or other fizzy drinks.
- Oranges pair well with ginger. Add both to stir-fried pork or chicken with spinach or kale.
- Add orange juice as a flavoring to mashed sweet potatoes or winter squash.
- Use orange juice instead of broth or wine to moisten stuffing.
- Mix orange juice with honey and ginger to make a glaze for turkey or chicken.

PIZZA

Italians love pizza. Italians also have a lower incidence of cancers of the digestive tract than neighboring nations where pizza is not a national dish. Could there be a relationship between the two?

That's what researchers in Milan wanted to find out when they conducted a meta-analysis of the dietary habits of 38,000 northern Italians over a span of 19 years. They discovered that, yes indeed, pizza fanatics had a lower rate of **colorectal**, **esophageal**, **laryngeal**, **oral cavity** and **pharyngeal cancers** than their countrymen who ate the least pizza. A second study of 4,999 Italians found similar results.

The researchers noted, however, they did not find a relationship between eating pizza and hormone-related cancers, including **prostate cancer**, which made them conjecture that there could be something other than pizza creating the anti-cancer effect. For example, tomatoes and tomato products, which are rich in lycopene and a key ingredient in pizza, are associated with a reduced risk of prostate cancer.

So, what's the bottom line? Can eating pizza really offer protection against cancer? Perhaps. The researchers conceded that Italians who eat a lot of pizza could also follow other healthy dietary and lifestyle practices that contribute to their lower cancer risk.

So, can pizza be part of an anti-cancer diet? Absolutely, as long as you eat pizza like it is made in Italy.

In the Kitchen with Pizza

Greasy pizza smothered with double cheese with a thick "Chicago style" crust is not the way to go. Traditional Italian pizza is made on a thin crust, like a flatbread, which is sometimes mixed with cancer-fighting rosemary. It is always made in a brick oven.

You will never find dry shredded mozzarella cheese on pizza in Italy. A true Italian pizza contains only fresh buffalo mozzarella cheese. It is also topped with olive oil, herbs and often, but not always, a thin layer of marinara sauce, and, of course, lots of chopped fresh garlic.

You don't have to make your own dough from scratch to imitate authentic Italian pizza. Make an individual pizza pie using good quality pita bread. To make a classic margherita pizza, drizzle the bread with olive oil, and cover with thinly sliced tomato or a thin layer of prepared marinara sauce. Slice and top with fresh buffalo mozzarella, garlic, and fresh basil. Bake in a 400°F oven for 10 minutes or until the cheese is melted and the crust crisp.

POMEGRANATE JUICE

If real men don't drink pomegranate juice, then real men are robbing their prostates of some very important protection.

More than a dozen studies have investigated the role of this curious-looking fruit in cancer prevention and the strongest evidence suggests that it helps fight **prostate cancer**. In one study, scientists from the University of California exposed pomegranate extract to highly aggressive prostate cancer cells in tissue cultures. They found that the extract slowed cancer growth and promoted cancer cell death.

In another study, the same researchers implanted two groups of mice with prostate cancer cells, but put only one group on a pomegranate diet. The mice that received water laced with pomegranate juice developed significantly smaller tumors than mice that didn't get any juice. In yet another study, researchers found that men with prostate cancer who drank pomegranate juice daily for 15 months had slower-growing tumors than men who did not drink the juice.

Pomegranate is rich in a number of polyphenols and researchers aren't sure yet which are playing the leading role in fighting cancer cells. Pomegranate contains at least four cancer-fighting nutrients: betulinic acid, genistein, ellagic acid, and ursolic acid. All have the ability to interfere with intracellular testosterone synthesis, a process that promotes cancer cell growth.

Other ongoing research is looking for a link between pomegranate and a reduced incidence of **breast**, **lung**, and **skin cancers**.

In the Kitchen with Pomegranate

If you've ever tasted grenadine, then you've already experienced pomegranate. Grenadine, a popular ingredient in mixed drinks, is sweetened and thickened pomegranate juice. However, it is not recommended as a substitute for the juice because it is laden with sugar. Pure pomegranate juice can be purchased at most supermarkets and health food stores. For something more exotic, however, buy a fresh pomegranate and sample the seeds in their pure naturalness.

Pomegranate is not valued for its pulp, but for its seed. The seeds encase almost the entire cavity of the fruit and look like deep red jewels encased in liquid. To open the fruit, score it with a knife, then break it apart or softly smack it against a hard surface to crack it open.

The seeds must then be extracted from the peel and internal white pulp membranes. This can be a bit tricky. The easiest way to do it is to put a bowl in the sink and fill it halfway with water. Submerge the broken fruit pieces in the bowl. The seeds will fall to the bottom and the pulp will float to the top. Simply scoop out the seeds and place them in a dry bowl.

The whole seeds can be eaten raw, though the watery seed casing, called the aril, is the desired part. The taste may differ from one fruit to the other, depending on the ripeness. The seeds are popular in Middle Eastern cuisine and are often dried and made into chutney and other types of relishes. Here are a few ideas to experiment with pomegranate on your own.

- Mix a few tablespoons of pomegranate seeds into homemade guacamole.
- Use pomegranate juice instead of wine or broth to deglaze a pan to make a gravy or sauce. It blends particularly well with chicken and pork.
- Sprinkle the seeds in fruit salad or a green salad.

• Make a fruit chutney by combining 3 cups of red raspberries, 1 cup of pomegranate juice, a half cup of sugar and a quarter cup of lime juice in a saucepan and simmer for about 20 minutes. Stir in a quarter cup of chopped cilantro and cool.

SHIITAKE MUSHROOMS

For something that thrives on the dead bark of Japanese forest trees, shiitake mushrooms are held in high regard in gourmet circles. They are also held in high regard in cancer research centers where scientists are investigating a special substance in shiitake mushrooms called lentinan that appears to be particularly resourceful at fighting cancer.

In one study, researchers injected lentinan directly into human **stomach cancer** cells in the test tube. What they saw was nothing short of amazing. The tumor sites developed special immune-fighting cells called reticular fibers that proliferated like mushrooms in dank, damp tree trunks. They also attracted T lymphocytes, another immune defender, to come to the aid of the reticular fibers. The onslaught caused the tumor-causing cell cluster to break up and self-destruct.

In another laboratory study on **breast cancer** tumors, researchers found lentinan fought back more than 50 percent of cells that were trying to colonize into tumors. Lentinan was even stronger at inhibiting malignant cells from spreading.

In yet another study, researchers wanted to find out how shiitake mushrooms would perform against **colon cancer** in mice. One group of mice was orally fed concentrated lentinan for seven days. The other group got no lentinan. On day eight all the mice were injected with human colon cancer cells. After one month, they measured the size of the tumors. They found tumor growth was significantly slower in the mice fed lentinan.

In the Kitchen with Shiitake Mushrooms

Shiitake mushrooms are expensive and are perishable. You can find them fresh or dried in Asian markets and most upscale supermarkets.

When buying fresh, look for mushrooms that are firm and plump and devoid of wet spots. They should be stored unwashed in the refrigerator and should keep for up to a week. To clean, simply wipe them with a damp paper towel or a mushroom brush. You don't want to rinse them, as they are very porous and will absorb moisture.

If you have a choice between buying fresh or dried, consider the dried. For one, they can be kept sealed for up to six months. More importantly, they have a more intense flavor and denser texture than fresh shiitakes.

To soften dried mushrooms, put them in just enough hot water to submerge them until they soften, about 30 minutes. Some cooks save the water and add it to soup broths and sauces. Finely chopped dried mushrooms contribute an earthy flavor to soups, stews, pasta and rice dishes. Add them to a wine sauce for meat or poultry.

Shiitake mushrooms are a signature ingredient in miso soup and are often included in Chinese stir-fries.

SOY FOODS

Some people consider soy an alternative food favored only by vegetarians and health nuts. Truth is, soy is so mainstream that it is almost impossible to avoid. Just take a look at the ingredient lists on the food packages in your pantry. Chances are you'll find soy in at least half of them. And that's good, because a few servings of soy a day can protect both men and women against hormone-related cancers.

Soy is rich in isoflavones, including daidzein, genistein, and equol, and is the richest source of phytoestrogens, which—as their name implies—are akin to the female hormone estrogen.

Female Friendly

Researchers have been looking for a link between soy consumption and reduced risk of **breast cancer** for years, though studies have been mixed. Nevertheless, statistics show that breast cancer rates are lowest in countries where soy is a dietary staple, most notably China, Korea, and Japan, and highest in developed nations, such as the United States, that aren't dependent on soy as a food supply. A more recent study of 73,223 adolescent and adult women in China may explain, at least in part, why findings are mixed. It appears that eating soy food has a significant impact on reducing the risk of getting breast cancer before menopause but not after. Also, greater benefits have been observed in women who started eating soy as a child. Why? Because phytoestrogens appear to act in humans the same way they behave in animals. When researchers fed the nutrient to young animals, they found that their mammary glands became more resistant to tumors.

Soy takes on extra significance for women who drink. Soy has been found to neutralize the toxic effects of alcohol (a risk factor of breast cancer), so even women who drink only moderately should take advantage of eating soy products no matter what their age.

Consuming soy foods also has been found to be

protective against **endometrial cancer,** which is linked to overweight and overproduction of estrogen. One study of 500 women in the San Francisco Bay area between the ages of 35 and 70 found that obese post-menopausal women eating the lowest amount of soy foods had the highest risk of all for endometrial cancer.

Most recently, researchers at Vanderbilt University School of Medicine found that consuming 10 grams of soy protein a day can reduce the risk of **colorectal cancer** in most menopausal women. Ten grams is equal to a half cup of tofu or edamame.

Soy is just as beneficial to men as it is to women. Incidence of **prostate cancer** is also lower in Asian countries than in the United States and other developed nations, and much of the credit goes to soy. One Japanese study of 43,509 men found the protective effect was strongest in men 60 and older. Isoflavones act the same way in men as they do in women—by altering the metabolism of estrogen. This, in turn, helps reduce testosterone levels. (Yes, men do manufacture some estrogen, just as women have some testosterone in their bodies.)

Other studies have linked consumption of soy foods for a reduced risk of **bladder**, **blood**, **lung**, and **stomach cancer**.

In the Kitchen with Soy Foods

Experts recommend getting a minimum of three to four servings of soy products a week and there is a diversity of ways to do so—without resorting to imitation hot dogs and burgers. Imitation means manufactured or processed, so these products are not all that good for you anyway. It's best to stick to the real thing, and there are plenty of options. Soy milk, soy flour, and soy oil are readily available for use in your own recipes.

Here are some ways to enjoy soy:

- Soybeans, better known as edamame, are popular these days and they make a great snack. They can be found packaged, ready to pop in your mouth, at most supermarkets.
- If you've tried tofu and didn't like it, try again. Tofu is the chameleon of soy and has the ability to take on the flavor of other foods it mingles with in a dish. Just don't cook it too long. The isoflavones in tofu deteriorate when heated, so add it to a dish in the last few minutes.
- Bean sprouts have mild flavor and good crunch, making them a great addition to sandwiches and salads.
- Use soymilk as a substitute for cow's milk in your coffee or tea.
- Substitute half soy flour for regular flour in recipes.
- Infuse soy oil with your favorite herbs and use for dipping bread.
- Add garlic to the infused oil, heat it gently, and use it to dress pasta.
- Use soybean oil to stir-fry meats and vegetables. For a little flavor, add a splash of sesame oil.
- Miso soup is popular and deceivingly simple. Miso can be found in packets and is as easy to make as other instant soup.
- When checking out products in the supermarket, look for soy on the label. If it's listed in the first three ingredients, it will help stoke your soy intake.

SPINACH

Spinach is the superman of cancer warfare. It acts like a heat-seeking missile at targeting and terminating damaged cells that would otherwise turn into tumors. All its strength comes from a unique profile of phytochemicals called phenols that help protect you from cancer.

Yes, broccoli contains more phenols than any other vegetable, but the phenols in spinach work the hardest. In fact, spinach's anti-cancer activity is so impressive that researchers wish they could bottle it so we could swig it down, just like Popeye. How's that for an endorsement to eat your spinach!

Scientists have developed spinach extracts to test its anti-cancer strength, and what they've found to date is very promising. Test tube and animal studies have found that spinach can win a battle at the cellular level and knock back the most life-threatening cancers, including **breast**, **colon**, **lung**, **ovarian**, **prostate**, **skin** and **stomach cancers**.

In one example, scientists in Japan purified a major component of spinach and tested it in mice in various stages of colon cancer. In one study, the extract inhibited the DNA damage that leads to cancer. In another it decreased the size of a cancerous tumor by 56 percent in just two weeks—and without any side effects.

So, how does this translate to humans eating the real thing? Researchers in North Carolina found out during a breast cancer study that was looking for an association between reduced risk and intake of vegetables rich in vitamin A and beta-carotene, such as spinach and carrots. After analyzing the diets of 12,949 women for three years they found that women who ate the most spinach and carrots had the lowest rate of breast cancer compared to women who ate the least.

In another study, researchers calculated the flavonoid intake in 66,940 women enrolled in the long-term Nurses' Health Study and found that those who ate foods containing the most active compounds had a 40 percent reduced risk of ovarian cancer.

In the Kitchen with Spinach

Whether fresh or frozen, spinach is on the adventurous cook's dream team. It is one of the most versatile vegetables and is equally delicious raw or cooked. It can find a place in just about any type of dish. It fits in an omelet at breakfast, as a filling for lasagna, and as a topping on pasta or pizza. It can be combined with eggs, honey, almonds, and spices as a filling for a dessert tart or flan.

It's also durable. Spinach retains much of its cancer-scavenging activity during cooking, but microwaving retains the most. Wilting it briefly in a sauté pan and using it in a stir-fry actually increases its nutritional power.

When buying spinach, look for leaves and stems that are crisp and deep green in color. Signs of yellow or wilting mean that they are past their prime. Refrigerate spinach unwashed in a loose plastic bag. Once exposed to water it can spoil quickly. This includes cooked spinach.

When you are ready to use spinach, wash it thoroughly, as it tends to collect sand and soil. If you are buying farm-fresh spinach, you will need to wash it very well. Trim the stems from the leaves and put them in a large bowl of tepid water. Swish the leaves around to dislodge the dirt. You might have to repeat the process several times.

SWEET POTATOES

The saying *beauty is more than skin deep* may be an old cliché, but there is no better way to describe the sweet potato. This dirt-groveling, oddly shaped tuber is no beauty but what lies beneath the skin is about as good as it gets.

The sweet potato contains a whole cast of anti-cancer nutrients, including vitamins A and C, folate, zinc, and a swarm of antioxidant phytonutreints too numerous to mention. But the sweet potato is best known for being the richest source of beta-carotene. At least 70 studies have found that cancer is higher among people who don't eat enough produce containing beta-carotene. A sweet potato is so rich in beta-carotene that you'd have to eat 23 cups of broccoli to get the same amount found in one average sweet potato.

And there's more. A sweet potato has virtually no fat and is full of fiber, both important anti-cancer qualities, especially when it comes to reducing the risk of **colon cancer**.

Even the skin of the potato is good for you. Like many fruits, sweet potato skin contains anthocyanins, rare phytochemicals with unique cancer-fighting ability. The Center for Science in the Public Interest says that the most important dietary change a person can make is to eat sweet potatoes on a regular basis.

In the Kitchen with Sweet Potatoes

It's in everyone's best interest to make sweet potatoes more than a holiday tradition. It's easy to do, too, because sweet potatoes are available year round and are very durable.

When buying, look for firm and heavy sweet potatoes that do not have any cracks, bruises, or soft spots. Store them in a cool, dark place with plenty of ventilation. In the summer, this could be the garage or cellar. Keep them out of the refrigerator, because the cold will alter the taste.

Sweets are conducive to all types of cooking methods except boiling, which robs much of their nutritional content. When it comes to cooking ideas, sweet potatoes are more versatile than white potatoes. Here are a few ideas:

- Bake sweet potatoes and acorn squash until just soft. Scoop out the flesh from each and mash together along with maple syrup, a little milk, cinnamon, and nutmeg.
- Puree cooked sweets in a blender with a ripe banana. Top with chopped walnuts and bake until heated through.
- Cut into chunks and add to stews and vegetable soups or scatter them around the baking pan when roasting chicken.
- Slice them as you would French fries and bake them in the oven until crisp.

TOMATOES

Tomatoes are the crown jewel of men's health, thanks to a rare substance called lycopene that has been found to be the great defender of the prostate.

Tomatoes gained status as a super food more than a decade ago when scientists found that tomatoes are a rare super source of lycopene, a carotenoid with an unusual ability to help stop **prostate cancer** before it can even get started. More than 85 percent of the lycopene that exists in food is found in the tomato. It's a true heavyweight, too, for it increases in strength when tomatoes get cooked into pasta sauce, bottled as ketchup, or laced over pizza dough with a heavy dose of olive oil.

These days you can't find a better refuge for the prostate than a good Italian restaurant. Hundreds of studies have been conducted on the virtues of lycopene, including many on humans. The vast majority name lycopene a leading defensive weapon against prostate cancer.

An analysis of 21 studies on lycopene and prostate cancer concluded that eating tomatoes, especially cooked tomatoes, is a safeguard against the disease. They found that men who ate raw tomatoes had an 11 percent reduced risk, but men who ate cooked tomatoes had a 19 percent reduced risk. Even one serving a day of raw tomatoes contributed to a reduced risk of 3 percent.

The prostate trials prompted more studies to find out if lycopene is resistant to other cancers as well, though results have been inconsistent. The strongest evidence suggests that it may be protective against **colorectal cancer**. When researchers compared blood levels of lycopene in people with colon cancer, they found levels 35 percent lower than in people who did not have any precancerous or cancerous polyps. Another study found that lycopene appeared to reduce the incidence of **pancreatic cancer** by 31 percent.

Most recently, research at Ohio State University suggests that it is not lycopene alone, but rather the total nutritional characteristics of tomato that make it such a cancer-fighting warrior.

"Our findings strongly suggest that risks of poor dietary habits cannot be reversed simply by taking a pill," commented Steven Clinton, one of the Ohio State researchers. "If we want the health benefits of tomatoes, we should eat tomatoes or tomato products and not rely on lycopene supplements alone."

In the Kitchen with Tomatoes

There are tomatoes, and then there are *real* tomatoes. Hothouse tomatoes, the kind most often found in supermarkets even during peak growing season, are pale and bland compared to the rich, juicy flavor of deep red ripe tomatoes grown on the vine. They make the best eating for sandwiches, gazpacho soup, and salads.

But even if you can't get the best that summer has to offer, there is plenty of opportunity to enjoy tomatoes all year round. Tomatoes come in dozens of varieties. Here are some tips on getting the most nutritional value from eating tomatoes:

- Several studies found that cooking tomatoes increases lycopene's anti-cancer activity. One study found that cooking tomatoes in olive oil makes their cancer-fighting power even more potent.
- Studies found that whole canned tomatoes contain more lycopene that chopped tomatoes. So even if your recipe calls for chopped and seeded tomatoes, buy whole tomatoes and do the chopping and seeding yourself.
- Tomato paste contains more lycopene than whole tomatoes. Tomato paste is usually used in small amounts, so buy it in a tube so it doesn't go to waste. It can last in the refrigerator for months.
- Take advantage of the nutritional value of tomato paste by using it as a thickener in soups and stews.
- Perk up commercial pasta sauce by adding 2 cups of fresh or canned chopped tomatoes while it is cooking.
- Take advantage of tomatoes in season by making large batches of sauces and freezing them in family-size containers.
- Perk up the taste of winter tomatoes by adding lots of herbs and spices. Oregano, marjoram, basil, and tarragon are naturals in tomato sauces.
- Gazpacho, a cold raw soup based on tomatoes, is a natural during the summer. All you need to do

is puree tomatoes, tomato juice, cucumbers, bell
peppers, red onions, garlic, spices, salt and a little
olive oil in a food processor and serve.
• All kinds of tomato products will give you a protective dose of lycopene. Take advantage of ketchup,
juice, soup, sauce and paste.

WALNUTS

Walnuts have been widely studied for their ability to
protect against heart disease, and now a new study
shows that they may be protective against **breast cancer**, as well. Walnuts contain a variety of healthful nutrients, including omega-3 fatty acids, ellagic acids, and
phytosterols—all substances with anti-cancer activity.

Researchers from Marshall University in Huntington,
West Virginia, wanted to find out if a typical snack-size
serving of walnuts possessed enough power to resist
cancer. For the study, the researchers fed breast cancer-
induced mice the human equivalent of 2 ounces of walnuts a day. Another group of mice received no walnuts.
"These laboratory mice typically have one hundred percent tumor incidence at five months," explained Elaine
Hardman, Ph.D., one of the researchers. "Walnut consumption delayed these tumors by three weeks." Hardman said the experiment demonstrates that eating
walnuts significantly decreased breast tumor incidence,
the number of glands with a tumor, and tumor size. The
most benefit came from the omega-3 fatty acids.

"With dietary interventions you see multiple mechanisms when working with the whole food," said
Dr. Hardman. "It is clear that walnuts contribute to a
healthy diet that can reduce breast cancer."

The best way to get more walnuts in your diet is to
eat them as a snack.

WATER

Water does much more than keep you hydrated. It is a natural detoxifier that helps your liver rid your body of potentially harmful carcinogens by flushing them out of your system. Natural doctors recommend drinking at least 8 glasses of water a day as a natural body purifier.

A three-day juice fast is an alternative form of detoxification, but this is not recommended for everyone, especially if you are not in good health. Water, however, is essential.

Drink 8 to 10 8-ounce glasses a day. This can include fresh fruit juices.

WATERCRESS

Watercress is the Cinderella of the cruciferous family. At one time, its importance was relegated to tea sandwiches, garnish, and the occasional soup until a few years ago when researchers found that this wilting violet can stand up against cancer as well as hardier members of the clan, such as cabbage and broccoli.

In one of the few human studies on the nutritional impact of watercress, researchers put 60 healthy young men and women on a daily diet that included watercress for eight weeks. They found it reduced DNA damage by 23 percent. Researchers believe this was due to its rich content of beta-carotene and lutein, two antioxidants with demonstrated anti-cancer activity. After the eight weeks, the volunteers' lutein levels had increased 1,000 percent and beta-carotene levels were up 33 percent.

"Population studies have shown links between higher intakes of cruciferous vegetables like watercress, and a reduced risk of a number of cancers," commented Ian Rowland, one of the researchers. "What makes this study unique is it involves people eating watercress in easily achievable amounts."

The achievable amount used in the study was 3 ounces a day.

Watercress also is rich in other cancer-fighting nutrients including vitamins A and C and calcium. But its real power may come from a tongue twister called phenethyl isothiocyanate, a much-studied, highly reactive molecule with numerous anti-cancer activities, including the ability to purge the body of carcinogens, reduce the risk of genetic damage that can lead to cancer, and inhibit the growth of cancerous cells.

In the Kitchen with Watercress
Watercress is an aquatic plant that takes special care to grow and ship. It is highly perishable, so make sure to use it within a day or two of purchasing. Buy only bunches that are green and that stand up on their stems. If they appear wilted or listing, they are beyond their prime.

For having such a tender image, watercress has a full-bodied taste that many favor over its garniture competitor, parsley. In addition to its well-known role as the star in English tea sandwiches, here are some other ideas:

- Use watercress as a substitute for spinach in omelets, dips, and soups.
- Pair it with oranges and red onion as a salad with ginger dressing.
- Pair it with cream cheese on a bagel.
- Chop it, sprinkle it with olive oil, and mash it into potatoes.
- Use it instead of lettuce on a chicken salad or tuna sandwich.
- Add it to other ingredients in gazpacho.

WHOLE GRAINS

If you eat daily from the fruits and vegetables recommended in this chapter, you'll make great strides in one of the major challenges of the Western diet—getting enough fiber.

The American diet is sorely lacking in fiber, a problem that started shortly after the Civil War when the steel roller made the refining of flour a cheap and easy process. When grains are processed, two of the three layers are removed—the bran and the germ, or, in other words, the fiber.

Fiber is essential to regularity. It is also essential to cancer prevention. A review of 16 years of studies on 20 different types of cancer found that overall cancer risk came down as consumption of whole grains increased. This was most noticeable for **colorectal cancer**. Conversely, they also observed that cancer rates increased in diets containing refined, rather than whole grains. This was most noticeable for **breast**, **colorectal**, **digestive tract**, and **endometrial cancer**s.

Eating fiber has the greatest impact on breast and colorectal cancers. When researchers looked at the fiber consumption of 35,972 women, they found that a diet rich in fiber from whole grains and fruit offered significant protection against breast cancer among pre-menopausal women. They found that eating 30 grams a day or more reduced risk by 52 percent.

In the Kitchen with Whole Grains

If you're like the typical American, you could stand to get more fiber in your diet. According to statistics, American men only get an average of 17.8 grams of fiber a day. Women get even less—an average of 13.6 grams. The American Cancer Society recommends a minimum of

25 grams of fiber a day. Here are ways you can increase your fiber intake.

- Apples and pears are rich sources of pectin, a special type of fiber that is associated with a reduced risk of **colorectal cancer**. Get pectin in your diet daily.
- Eat berries every chance you get. Not only are they super cancer fighters, but they are loaded with fiber.
- Eat a whole grain cereal for breakfast every day. Look for cereal that contains at least 3 grams of fiber per serving.
- Get white bread out of the house and only eat bread made from whole grains.
- Find a low-fat recipe for bran muffins and eat them as a snack.
- Popcorn is a great fiber-filled snack and a good substitute for chips and other salty snacks.

WINE

There is no room in an anti-cancer diet for hard liquor—but there can be an exception for wine. Though heavy consumption of alcohol is associated with an increased risk of certain cancers, several studies have found that modest consumption of wine can help prevent them.

What wine contains and hard liquor lacks are polyphenols. Wine contains more than 500 active substances, but researchers believe that one in particular is responsible for wine's anti-cancer qualities: resveratrol.

Resveratrol is a unique polyphenol that is concentrated in the skin and seeds of the grape. It is much more powerful as wine than grape juice because the fermenting process that turns grapes into wine concentrates and expands resveratrol.

Hundreds of studies have found that resveratrol has the ability to restore normal growth to precancerous tumor cells and counteract toxic substances in the body. Its ability to neutralize toxicity is the reason why wine has been found to be the only beverage that may help reduce the risk of **lung cancer**.

Researchers at Kaiser Permanente Southern California did an analysis of more than 20 studies on the association between alcohol and lung cancer. They found that drinking more than a glass or two a day of beer or hard liquor increased the risk of lung cancer by 20 to 30 percent in men, but moderate consumption of wine was protective against the disease in both men and women.

Why alcohol contributes to lung cancer is somewhat of a mystery, but there is an obvious reason why it can lead to **esophageal cancer**. The harsh chemicals that make up ethanol, the substance that creates the alcoholic effects of liquor, irritate the esophagus, which causes heartburn that can lead to a condition called Barrett's esophagus, a reflux condition that can lead to esophageal cancer. At least that's the experience for beer and hard liquor drinkers, but apparently not for wine drinkers.

Another study, also conducted by Kaiser Permanente, followed the drinking habits of 953 men and women in Northern California and found that modest wine consumption had a protective effect against Barrett's esophagus. Beer and spirits did not have the same effect. Studies in Australia and Ireland reported similar findings.

It's not clear why wine lowers the risk of Barrett's esophagus, but researchers figure the antioxidants in wine neutralize the damage created by reflux disease. People also tend to drink wine with food, which can also reduce the damaging effects.

Though drinking is associated with an increased risk of **breast cancer**, resveratrol has been found to have an inhibiting effect on hormones found in cancerous breast cells.

Whatever wine's beneficial effects are, they are apparently long lasting, because researchers at Yale School of Public Health found that years of wine drinking can help improve the prognosis for people who get cancer. At least that was the experience for a group of women with **non-Hodgkin's lymphoma**. Among the 546 women in the study, lymphoma patients who had been consuming wine for at least 25 years had a 25 to 35 percent reduced risk of death, relapse, or developing a secondary cancer than non-wine drinkers.

"This conclusion is controversial, because excessive drinking has a negative social and health impact, and it is difficult to define what is moderate and what is excessive," noted researcher Xuesong Han. "However, we are continually seeing a link between wine and positive outcomes in many cancers."

There is another theory associated with the protective effects of drinking wine—lifestyle. Wine drinkers tend to lead healthier lives and have a better diet than people who prefer beer or hard liquor. Statistics show that wine drinkers do not eat a lot of red meat or saturated fat, are generally thin, and tend to be non-smokers. They also drink wine as part of a meal. If you want to drink wine as part of an anti-cancer diet, follow these guidelines:

- Drink in moderation—that's one 5-ounce glass of wine a day for women and two for men.
- Drink red over white. Resveratrol is concentrated in the skin of the grape, which is peeled to make white wine. The skin is retained in manufacturing red wine.

YOGURT

Probiotics do not sound very appetizing, but they are very important to your health. They are also a hedge against **colorectal cancer**.

Probiotics are live antimicrobial substances found in certain brands of yogurt that are specifically designed to improve and maintain health in the lower digestive system. The action comes from two specific species called lactobacillus and bifidobacterium.

Research shows that probiotics protect against colon cancer in several ways. They help alleviate intestinal inflammation (and chronic inflammation leads to cancer), they detoxify acids in foods that irritate the intestine or colon and cause inflammation, and they also suppress the growth of bacteria in the intestines that attract carcinogens.

In the Kitchen with Yogurt

Try to get one cup of probiotic yogurt daily for intestinal health. Look for yogurt containing at least 4 billion organisms of the friendly bacteria per serving. Your best bet to save calories and fat is to purchase plain, low-fat yogurt, then dress it up by adding chopped fruit, nuts, and herbs or spices, such as fresh mint and basil leaves. You can also stir it into breakfast cereal in place of milk, and add it to a fruit smoothie.

CHAPTER 5

Supplements that Help Fight Cancer

The shelves of health food stores and pharmacies are filled with scores of natural substances claiming to provide protection against cancer. Sifting through the array of vitamins, herbs, and other substances can be mind-boggling if you don't know *exactly* what you are looking for.

Also, you may well wonder, is the nutritional supplement going to offer the same protection as the nutrient found in the food? If so, what is the right amount to take? How much of the nutrient can the body absorb? And, how safe is it to take herbs or supplemental natural substances manufactured by the body that are not found in food?

The FDA doesn't offer much help. Federal regulations for dietary supplements are very different from those for prescription and over-the-counter drugs. For example, a dietary supplement manufacturer does not have to prove a product's safety and effectiveness before it is marketed.

Then there's the very real possibility that the nutrient found in a particular food helps protect against cancer, because it gets a big boost from other substances in the food. Taking the nutrient alone could offer little or no protection at all.

On the flip side, supplements can be very beneficial because they can also offer therapeutic amounts of a nutrient or herb that is impossible to get from a normal diet. Resveratrol, the antioxidant that makes red wine a cancer fighter, is the perfect example. You would have to drink thousands of glasses of wine to get the same amount of resveratrol found in just one supplement. Another example is blackberry powder. It would be impossible to eat enough berries in a day to come close to getting the nutritive value found in a teaspoon of powder.

This chapter should help dissolve any quandaries you might have about supplements and cancer prevention, because it features only supplements that have been scientifically demonstrated to have anti-cancer activity. Only you and your health care provider, however, can decide which are appropriate to take, and that should depend on your current state of health, your personal dietary habits, the prescription medications that you are taking, and your risk factors.

There are several caveats concerning dietary supplements that you need to consider before going to the health food store:

Before you begin taking supplements, discuss them with your doctor. This is especially important if you are taking medication for a health condition, or if you are pregnant, breastfeeding, or planning to become pregnant.

Just because it's natural does not mean it's safe. Supplements can be toxic at high levels just like drugs. Only take the amount specified on the bottle or recommended by your doctor. And make sure the supplement or supplements you are planning to take are compatible with your prescription medication. Supplements can interact with other supplements or medications in unfavorable ways, either by neutralizing, enhancing, or diminishing their strength.

Supplements are not intended to replace medication you are currently taking. Do not go off any medication or change dosage without the knowledge and consent of your doctor. Certain supplements can render certain medications ineffective, especially drugs for serious illnesses, such as cancer, high blood pressure, and cholesterol.

Cancer patients should be extra cautious. If you are taking chemotherapy drugs or other cancer drugs, do not take any supplements without the knowledge and consent of your oncologist. Certain supplements can affect cancer drugs in either a positive or negative way. For example, a recent study found that the active ingredient in green tea and green tea extract can make chemotherapy drugs for lymphoma ineffective.

Keep supplements in a safe place. This means out of the reach of children. Supplements should be stored in a dry, cool place and away from direct light, meaning *not* in the bathroom or near the kitchen sink. Throw away any supplements that are past their expiration date.

Be alert to side effects. Supplements can have side effects even if taken in recommended dosages. This can include an allergic reaction. If you experience any of these symptoms, discontinue use and seek emergency treatment, if needed:

• Hives
• Itchy or swollen skin

- Difficulty breathing
- Tightness in the chest

Many nutrients are under investigation for their potential role in helping to fight cancer. These 26 are among the most promising.

AGED GARLIC EXTRACT

Garlic ranks high as a cancer-protecting food, so if you don't get garlic in your diet every day, you might want to consider taking garlic capsules. It provides all the anti-cancer protection of fresh garlic, without the unwanted reminder of your last (or yesterday's) meal.

If you want to get the most from garlic cloves, go for aged garlic extract (AGE). Hundreds of studies suggest it's even better than the real thing.

AGE is extracted from fresh bulbs that have been left to sit at room temperature for 20 months, just enough time for the anti-cancer properties to multiply. During this aging time, harsh, unstable compounds gradually convert into stable health-promoting substances. AGE contains concentrated allicin, the substance that gives the herb its special cancer-preventing qualities. Aged garlic also contains flavonoids and the mineral selenium. In fact, one study found that the organosulfurs and selenium in AGE work better to guard against cancer than eating garlic or taking a selenium supplement alone.

Men at risk for **prostate cancer** might want to considered aged garlic. Two compounds unique to aged garlic, S-allyl cysteine and S-allyl mercaptocysteine, have been found to inhibit the growth of human prostate cells by 80 percent, according to one study. These compounds also have been found to help fight the damage from UV rays that leads to **skin cancer**. Other studies showed that S-allyl mercaptocysteine helps stop the growth of **breast**, **colon**, and **leukemia cancer** cells. It also reduced colon cancer cell growth by 71 percent.

How Much to Take

The recommended dosage is 300 to 450 milligrams twice a day. AGE is generally considered safe, but there is a risk of side effects including bad breath, nausea, vomiting, and nosebleed. If you experience any symptoms, stop taking the supplement and see your doctor, if necessary.

ASTRAGALUS

Ayurvedic doctors have used this ancient herb, which goes by the name *huang qi* in China, as a healing tonic for centuries. Today it is playing an important role in cancer treatment.

More than 30 studies involving nearly 3,000 cancer patients found that when astragalus was used in combination with chemotherapy, it reduced tumors more effectively than when cancer drugs were used alone. It also helped improve survival rates. The studies, all conducted in China, found the herb most beneficial in fighting **colorectal cancer**.

Astragalus complements chemotherapy because of its ability to mobilize natural killer cells in the immune system.

How Much to Take

The recommended dosages to boost the immune system and prevent cancer is 1,000 milligrams a day. Anyone who has cancer and is undergoing chemotherapy should take the herb only after consulting with an oncologist.

BETA-CAROTENE

Beta-carotene has been synonymous with cancer prevention for decades. Back in the 1980s, after a number of studies found that it helped reduce the risk of lung cancer, smokers started popping beta-carotene like happy pills in the hope that that they could avoid cancer. Only it didn't happen. Lung cancer rates continued to rise.

More recently, similar studies on beta-carotene's ability to reduce the risk of cancer have been mixed. Two studies actually found that taking beta-carotene supplements *increased* cancer risk for smokers and workers exposed to secondhand smoke. In other studies on similar groups of people, beta-carotene did not appear to make a difference one way or the other. And yet other studies continue to show a reduced risk for **cervical** and **prostate cancers** in people taking supplemental beta-carotene.

Over the years beta-carotene has been found to be protective against other cancers, as well. For example, doctors in Italy reviewed 16 years' worth of beta-carotene studies and found that the nutrient is effective against **breast**, **colorectal**, **esophageal**, **oral** and **pharyngeal cancers.**

Beta-carotene is a highly active antioxidant belonging to a group of nutrients called carotenoids. Hopes were originally quite high in the nutritional fight against cancer as a result of evidence showing that people with lower levels of dietary carotenoids—meaning they didn't eat a lot of dark green and orange fruits and vegetables—had higher rates of lung cancer. Conversely, other data showed that high dietary intake of beta-carotene was associated with a reduced risk of cancer.

So, what gives?

Smokers Beware

The fly in the vitamin jar, it now seems, is tobacco. It appears that smokers who are longtime users of beta-carotene are actually putting themselves at risk for lung cancer. The indictment came in 2009 with the results of a large-scale study that found smokers who took beta-carotene and other lung-protecting vitamins were at a higher risk for developing lung cancer than the general public. The study followed the supplement habits of 77,000 Americans, ages 56 to 70, for 10 years and matched it against lung cancer data from a national cancer registry.

"The risk increased the longer the person had taken the supplements," reported lead researcher Jessie Satia, Ph.D., associate professor of epidemiology and nutrition at the University of North Carolina. "The amount of time the person took supplements seemed to have a greater effect than the dose. Even a modest dose, if taken for a long time, can increase the risk of lung cancer, especially among smokers." The other "at-risk vitamins" include retinol, lutein and lycopene.

This was not an isolated study, either. A study of male smokers over age 40 in the Netherlands found that beta-carotene supplementation not only increased the risk of lung cancer but also increased the risk of recurrence and death.

Taking beta-carotene also was found to reduce the effectiveness of cancer therapies in smokers. Netherlands researchers reported that drinking alcohol washed away any possible cancer-preventive effects from taking beta-carotene.

How Much to Take

Cancer experts generally agree that beta-carotene is a fine supplement to take for cancer prevention, *if* you are not a smoker. Beta-carotene has no known side effects and is well tolerated at high doses. The suggested daily dose is 2,500 IU. Experts suggest, however, that the best way to get beta-carotene is to load up on it through diet. These are some excellent sources of beta-carotene.

- Apricots
- Broccoli
- Butternut squash
- Carrots
- Green leafy vegetables
- Mango
- Papaya
- Pumpkin
- Sweet potatoes

BLACK COHOSH

Say black cohosh, think pink ribbons.

This herb, rooted in ancient lore, goes back to the early Indians, who used it as an aid during childbirth. In modern times it became a well-known aid in helping women control hot flashes and other side effects of menopause. Now, doctors believe it might help *prevent* breast cancer.

In the past, black cohosh was considered a cancer risk for the same reason it is a friend to women in menopause. The herb emits estrogen-like signals that are strong enough to quell hot flashes, but apparently not strong enough to activate breast cancer cells, and estrogen is known to increase the risk of breast cancer. However, preliminary research actually shows that black cohosh may decrease this risk. Doctors at the University of Pennsylvania School of Medicine studied more than 2,500 women and found that those who took black cohosh had a 61 percent *lower* risk of developing breast cancer.

Though black cohosh supplements are not yet recommended as an anti-cancer supplement, women should feel comfortable taking it for menopause without worrying about increasing their cancer risk. Women who are at increased risk for breast cancer, however, should discuss taking the herb with their doctor.

BLACK CUMIN OIL

The oil from the Indian spice *Nigella stavia* possesses a substance called thymoquinone that appears to have potent anti-cancer properties. Thymoquinone is an active antioxidant that may stimulate natural killer cells in the immune system to detect and destroy cancer cells. It's now being tested on at least two continents for its potential to both prevent and treat cancer.

Test tube studies in Beirut found thymoquinone was potent enough to kill cancer-forming cells that lead to **colon cancer**. They also found that it can keep tumors in the colon from growing. More recently, researchers at Jefferson Medical College in Philadelphia found that thymoquinone reduced the size of tumors by 67 percent in test animals induced with **pancreatic cancer**.

Jefferson doctors believe that the herb is a beneficial cancer preventative, especially for people with chronic pancreatitis, an inflammation that can lead to cancer, and for those at high risk for cancer. Other research has found the herb to be effective against **leukemia** and **prostate cancers**.

How Much to Take

"The herb and oil are safe when used moderately, and have been used for thousands of years without reported toxic effects," report the Jefferson researchers. The seeds can be used as a culinary spice or the oil can be used medicinally. Take the oil according to package directions.

BLACK RASPBERRY POWDER

Berries are *so* good, you might wonder why anyone would want to sacrifice a delectable taste in exchange for taking a supplement. Well, here's why: There is more cancer-fighting protection in less than a teaspoon of black raspberry extract than you can get from eating a pound of the real thing.

Sold as a powder or extract, supplemental black raspberry is a concentrated source of the freeze-dried berry, one of the most potent natural foods with anti-cancer properties. "You'd have to eat about a pound of black raspberries *every day* to get the same effect," says Gary D. Stoner, Ph.D., of Ohio State University and a leading researcher on black raspberries and cancer. "The freeze-drying process concentrates the active compounds in the berries about tenfold because berries are about ninety percent water."

Researchers still aren't sure of all their anti-cancer nutrients, but black raspberries stand out among all other berries as the richest sources of anthocyanins, cancer-fighting compounds concentrated in the skin.

In experiments at Ohio State University, Dr. Anne VanBuskirk found that freeze-dried black raspberries applied directly to the skin can help heal lesions that can lead to **skin cancer**. Dr. Susan Mallery found that a black raspberry gel had the same effect when applied to mouth sores in people at high risk for **oral cancer**. Taken internally, it can be protective against the toxic effects of tobacco that lead to **esophageal cancer**.

Dr. Stoner believes freeze-dried powder made from several different berry types can offer potentially life-saving protection to certain people at high risk for cancer. This includes people with:

- an inherited genetic defect that puts them at risk;
- higher-than-average exposure to known carcinogens, such as tobacco;
- premalignant lesions in the colon, esophagus and mouth or on the skin;
- non-malignant skin cancer lesions; and
- a risk for cancer recurrence.

How to Get Berry Powder

There are many ways to take berry powder, including dissolving it in water or juice, adding it to a smoothie or sprinkling it on cereal. Extract calls for taking about several drops a day under the tongue or dissolved in water.

Both powders and extracts can be found in some health food stores and are also sold online.

CALCIUM

For decades, women have been cautioned to protect their bones with calcium. Now, there is another reason to take a calcium supplement every day. A major population study of nearly half a million people found that calcium helps protect both men and women from many types of cancer, most particularly **colorectal cancer**.

It's advice that should be easy to swallow because the amount of calcium you need to get extra cancer protection is the same amount everyone over age 50 should get to protect their bones—around 1,200 milligrams a day.

The National Cancer Institute officially endorsed calcium supplementation as an anti-cancer strategy in 2009 after reviewing the results of a study that followed the food and supplement habits of 293,907 men and 198,903 women for seven years. All were cancer-free at the beginning of the study. At the end of the study, 36,965 cancer cases were identified in men and 16,605 in women. In women, the researchers found that calcium helped reduce the risk for **all forms of cancer**, but in men the impact was only noticed for **colorectal cancer**.

The women who consumed the most calcium (1,881 milligrams a day) had a 23 percent lower incidence of cancer than the women who consumed the least (494 milligrams a day). Risk reduction, however, leveled off at around 1,300 milligrams a day. In men, calcium intake is correlated with a reduced risk of **cancers involving the digestive system**. Men who consumed the most calcium (around 1,530 milligrams a day) had a 16 percent lower risk than men who consumed the least (526 milligrams).

Another smaller observational study suggests that taking aspirin with selenium could enhance calcium's effects against colorectal cancer.

How Much to Take

The study measured calcium intake from both food and a supplement. So, if you're looking for the same kind of protection, you should also be sure to eat calcium-rich foods. Dairy products are the richest source of calcium. You can get 1,200 milligrams a day by eating three cups of low-fat or non-fat dairy products daily. And here's the healthy kicker. Low- and no-fat dairy foods are higher in calcium than full-fat products. Other sources include:

Food	Amount	Milligrams
Milk, evaporated skim	1 cup	580
Sardines, with bones	3 ounces	372
Collard greens, cooked	1 cup	355
Yogurt	1 cup	272
Turnip greens, cooked	1 cup	252
Calcium-fortified fruit juice	1 cup	300
Milk, skim or 1%	1 cup	246
Milk, whole	1 cup	238
Buttermilk	1 cup	232
Salmon, with bones	3 ounces	167
Cottage cheese	½ cup	160
Broccoli	1 stalk	158
Almonds	2 ounces	132
Cheese, cheddar	1 cubic inch	129
Tofu	3.5 ounces	128

CAUTION: Men who have or are at risk for prostate cancer should not take calcium supplements without consulting with their doctor. Some studies have linked excess consumption of supplements and food containing calcium to an increase in prostate cancer.

CONJUGATED LINOLEIC ACID

Moo-ve over, Omega-3s, and make room for another helpful fatty acid. Conjugated linoleic acid, better known as CLA, is "good fat" joining the list of possible cancer fighters.

CLA is a group of 13 isomers (compounds with the same molecular profile but with different structures) that is best known as a weight-loss aid. Animal studies, however, have found that these isomers have anti-cancer and antioxidant properties that may help prevent and reduce tumors for several types of cancer including **melanoma**, **breast**, **colorectal**, **lung**, **prostate**, and **stomach cancers**.

CLA is not manufactured in the body. Its only source is the fat in dairy products and animals fed on grass, such as cows, goats, lambs, and deer. CLA was pushed as a weight-loss aid after animal studies found that it can help reduce body fat, especially around the abdomen, without losing lean muscle—and without changing dietary habits. This has positive implications for cancer prevention as well, because abdominal fat is a risk factor for cancer. How effective it really is as a weight-loss aid, however, is debatable. Nevertheless, its potential to fight cancer is being taken seriously. Noted one group of Argentine researchers, "CLAs are the only natural fatty acids accepted by the National Academy of Sciences of the USA as exhibiting consistent anti-tumor properties at levels as low as one-quarter to one percent of total fats."

What This Means to You

Even researchers who have found positive results in CLA's ability to fight cancer fall short of recommending supplements for across-the-board use. For one, there is the belief among some that CLA in animal products is superior to man-made synthetic CLA. Also, CLA supplements are expensive, mostly due to their promotion as a weight-loss aid.

Now the good news. You don't need to get a lot of CLA in your diet to reap its benefits. You'll get the most

CLA from grass-fed beef, lamb, and raw milk and cheese products, but you will also find some in regular milk, eggs, lean meat, and small amounts of cheese. If you decide you want extra CLA, it is sold as a soft gel supplement. Recommended dosage is 750 milligrams one to three times a day.

CURCUMIN

"Indian gold" is turning out to be more precious than 24-carat gold when it comes to both preventing and treating cancer.

"Whenever anybody asks me what supplement to take to prevent cancer, curcumin is *the* one," says Bharat B. Aggarwal, Ph.D., professor and chief of the Cytokine Research Center at the University of Texas M.D. Anderson Cancer Center in Houston.

Curcumin is the active ingredient in turmeric, the brilliantly yellow spice reminiscent of gold dust—thus, its moniker. Turmeric is a culinary staple in India and is found in just about every dish that crosses the table. It's best known for giving curries their bright yellow hue.

Curcumin is a rare substance—it is found *only* in turmeric—and it is currently one of the big hopefuls of cancer research. More than 1,000 studies have demonstrated that curcumin has strong powers to help stop cancer.

How Curcumin Works

Studies show that curcumin is a rich antioxidant and anti-inflammatory substance that can arrest low-grade inflammation that damages cells. This is important because inflammation is a main pathway leading to cancer, explains Dr. Aggarwal. Curcumin's remarkable anti-inflammatory power comes from its ability to disarm many of the proteins that promote chronic inflammatory processes in the body.

Curcumin appears to possess all the desirable features of a modern miracle drug, says Dr. Aggarwal, who is one of the world's leading experts on curcumin and its role in disease.

Research demonstrates that curcumin can:

- suppress the activation of genes that trigger cancer;
- kill renegade cells that mutate into cancer;
- shrink tumor cells;
- prevent tumors from spreading to other organs; and
- enhance the cancer-destroying effects of chemotherapy and radiation.

To date, curcumin has exhibited some or all of these actions against at least 17 different cancers. There is no other natural substance that has been found to possess this degree of anti-cancer power. For example:

- Thirty-four patients with advanced **pancreatic cancer** (usually lethal within one year) were given high daily doses of curcumin. The spice slowed progression of the disease in 64 percent of them.
- Researchers at Rutgers University found that a combined regimen of curcumin and isothiocyanate (an anti-cancer compound found in cruciferous vegetables, such as cauliflower, cabbage, and kale) reversed the growth of prostate tumors in mice. "Eating vegetable curry a few times a month might help prevent **prostate cancer**," noted researcher Tony Kong, M.D.

- Researchers at Dr. Aggarwal's M.D. Anderson Cancer Center conducted studies in which they injected mice with substances that produced **skin cancer**. They then treated half the mice by putting curcumin in their chow and the other half by applying curcumin as a paste to the cancerous lesions. In both cases, curcumin halted the progression of the disease in a majority of mice.

- When researchers added curcumin to Taxol, a common chemotherapy drug for **breast cancer**, it not only enhanced the effects of the drug but also decreased its toxic side effects, making the chemotherapy regime more tolerable for the patients.

- UCLA researchers found that curcumin prevented formation of polyps that lead to a particularly aggressive form of hereditary **colon cancer**. In another study on colon cancer, daily doses of three grams of curcumin reduced the number of precancerous lesions.

- More than 100 women with precancerous cervical lesions were put on eight grams of curcumin daily for three months. Twenty-five percent of the women experienced a reduction in lesions that are a precursor to **cervical cancer**.

- Research studies at M.D. Anderson found that curcumin inhibited the proliferation of cancerous cells in patients with **multiple myeloma**, an incurable but treatable cancer that attacks plasma cells.

- Researchers in Taiwan found that curcumin has the ability to decrease invasive **lung cancer** cells and stop them from spreading. This is a promising breakthrough because lung cancer is often at an advanced metastatic stage when it is detected.

- In China, curcumin stopped the proliferation and

invasion of **stomach cancer** cells. "Overall, these results provided novel insights into the mechanisms of curcumin inhibition of gastric cancer cell growth and potential therapeutic strategies for gastric cancer," concluded the researchers.

And the list goes on. Curcumin has been found to be a winning warrior against many other cancers, including **bone**, **bladder**, **blood**, **esophagus**, **kidney** and **liver cancers**.

A Capsule a Day

Curcumin has an unblemished safety record. There have been no reported serious side effects and no toxicity from taking up to 16 grams of curcumin a day. In culinary terms, that would be like eating a cup of turmeric!

The good news is that you don't need to get anywhere near that much to experience the anti-cancer benefits of curcumin. In India, the typical person ingests about a *teaspoon* of turmeric daily, spread out over three meals—enough for Indians to enjoy a remarkably low incidence of cancer.

The recommended daily intake for cancer protection is one 500-milligram tablet a day. You can get even more by experimenting in Indian cooking, such as making curries and spice blends that include turmeric.

Turmeric is the only edible source of curcumin, so adding it to your diet will give you even more cancer protection. (Curry powder is no substitute, as it is actually a spice blend that *includes* turmeric.)

There are two kinds of turmeric and they are named after their places of origin—Alleppey and Madras. Alleppey is the better of the two because it contains almost double the curcumin found in Madras. It also has a deeper color (bright yellow) and a mellower flavor. It will keep in a dry, dark storage area for up to one year.

CAUTION: Be careful of spills. This goes for both curcumin capsules and turmeric. During ancient times, turmeric had a secondary use as a fabric dye to make colorful clothing for the rich. Stains can be difficult to get out of certain fabrics and fibers.

ELLAGIC ACID

When you indulge in a bowl of red raspberries, your body cells get a full-force injection of ellagic acid, a powerful polyphenol well known for its anti-cancer activities.

Red raspberries are the richest source of ellagic acid. Cup for cup, they possess more than twice as much as any other food. Unfortunately, eating raspberries or walnuts (they're a good source, too) every day to get the anti-cancer benefits of ellagic acid is hardly realistic for most people. For one, berries are hard to find out of season. Plus, berries and nuts are expensive. However, there are cancer experts who believe the body shouldn't go a day without an infusion of this important cancer protector.

The next best thing to a bowl full of berries? A supplement.

How It Works

Ellagic acid is a powerful polyphenol that acts as an antioxidant by defending body cells. Our cells are in a continual cycle of replication. Healthy cells have a life cycle of about 120 days. When they die, other healthy cells replace them. Damaged cells, however, do not always die. In fact, they can multiply. When this happens, one cell becomes two, two become four, and so on until they cluster into a tumor you eventually feel as a lump. Animal studies show that ellagic acid can target and kill damaged cells without harming healthy ones. It also goes after growing cell clusters and stops them dead.

Researchers have seen this action in **colorectal**, **esophageal**, **liver**, and **prostate cancer** cell lines. Other laboratory studies found that ellagic acid seems to reduce the effect of estrogen in promoting growth of **breast cancer** cells in tissue cultures. There are also reports that it may help the liver break down or remove some cancer-causing substances from the blood.

Virtually all the research on ellagic acid and cancer has been done on animals and it has yet to be seen if the same results will be found in human studies.

How Much to Take

Cancer specialists say that you should take ellagic acid in addition to, and not in lieu of, a healthy diet, *including* eating red raspberries and other sources of the antioxidant, such as strawberries, pomegranates, and walnuts.

You can buy ellagic acid as a supplement or powder. Dosages range from 25 milligrams twice a day up to 500 milligrams. Side effects are rare, but include upset stomach, nausea and vomiting.

Chief food sources of ellagic acid include:

- Cranberries
- Pomegranate seeds or juice
- Pecans
- Red raspberries
- Strawberries
- Walnuts

FISH OIL (OMEGA-3 FATTY ACIDS)

If you don't care for fish and don't eat it at least twice a week, then you should consider taking fish oil tablets as a buffer against cancer.

Fish oil supplements are a direct source of omega-3 fatty acids, important immune boosters that guard against a number of diseases, including cancer. Studies have found that taking omega-3 fatty acid supplements containing eicosapentaenoic acid (EPA) and docosahexaenoic acid (DHA) help reduce risk and even slow tumor growth in a variety of cancers, including **breast**, **colon**, **lung**, and **prostate cancers**. One study found it reduced the risk of **kidney cancer** in women. It has also been shown to improve immunity in people undergoing surgery for colon cancer.

Chemotherapy Friendly

People undergoing chemotherapy or radiation may benefit from supplementing their diet with omega-3 fatty acids (as long as their oncologist approves). Studies have found that omega-3s can help:

- enhance the effects of chemotherapy drugs and, thus, improve chances of a favorable outcome;
- diminish unpleasant side effects; and
- reduce the risk of the cancer coming back.

That's a big package of possibilities! The benefits have been seen in treatment for cancers of various sites, including **breast**, **colon**, **esophageal**, **lung**, and **prostate cancers**.

It's even more helpful if you've been eating fish as a part of your regular diet. One study of women taking Tamoxifen for breast cancer found that women who had higher levels of fatty acids in breast tissue—indicating a diet already high in omega-3s—had a better response to the drug.

In Japan, where a lot of fish is consumed, researchers found that a diet rich in omega-3 fatty acids helped strengthen the immune system in people undergoing chemotherapy for **esophageal cancer**. The study also found it reduced toxic side effects, such as diarrhea.

"In combination with standard treatment, supplementing the diet with fatty acids may be a nontoxic means to improve cancer treatment outcomes and may slow or prevent recurrence of cancer," reported researchers at Louisiana State University, who reviewed all the literature in relation to cancer treatment and omega-3 fatty acids. "Used alone, a supplement may be a useful alternative therapy for patients who are not candidates for standard toxic cancer therapies."

Making "Fish" Taste Better

Some people complain that they stopped taking fish oil because it gave them a fishy aftertaste. If you've had this experience, try these strategies recommended by the Mayo Clinic.

Swallow the capsule frozen. This slows the breakdown of fish oil in the stomach, often reducing fishy burps. It will not affect digestion or absorption of the supplement.

Take it with food. Take the capsule just before mealtime. The fish oil will mix with food in the stomach, which will buffer the odor.

Try an odorless supplement. Coated capsules actually pass through the stomach and dissolve in the intestines.

Switch brands. Some manufacturers make a pure

omega-3 fatty acid product that doesn't taste fishy, although it is likely to cost more than standard products.

Common Food Sources
Fish is the best source of omega-3, but you can also get it from these sources:

- Cod liver oil
- Flaxseed oil
- Linseed oil

Take a daily fish oil capsule containing a combined 1,500 to 2,000 milligrams of DHA and EPA.

FLAXSEED OIL
If you're not fond of fish *or* fish oil supplements, then you should get familiar with flax.

Flaxseed oil, like fish oil, is rich in omega-3 fatty acids, but that's only part of the reason why flaxseed is an important anti-cancer supplement. Flaxseed is the richest source of lignans, a type of phytoestrogen that has been found to slow the growth of **breast cancer** tumors and help prevent the disease from spreading. Animal research also has found that fortifying the diet with supplemental flaxseed can help guard against **prostate cancer** and **melanoma**.

In more recent preliminary research, scientists from South Dakota State University found evidence that taking flaxseed oil supplements may help prevent **colorectal cancer** and keep tumors from growing as quickly in people who get the disease. The experiment was conducted on a special strain of mice that developed spontaneous intestinal tumors due to gene mutation. Mice fed a diet supplemented with flaxseed oil and flaxseed meal developed 45 percent fewer tumors than mice fed the same diet without supplemental flaxseed. The tumors that did develop in the flaxseed-fed mice were also smaller in size.

How Much to Take

Flaxseed oil has a buttery, nutty taste and should be taken straight by the tablespoon. One to two tablespoons a day is recommended, based on weight. The rule of thumb is 1 tablespoon per 100 pounds.

The oil is fragile and can turn rancid if not stored properly. It poorly tolerates heat, light, and oxygen, so it should be kept in an opaque bottle in the refrigerator. Buy oil that is cold-pressed to help assure quality.

Flaxseed oil also comes in soft gel capsules. The recommended dosage is 1 to 2 capsules daily.

FOLIC ACID

Folate deficiency is the most common vitamin deficiency in the United States, affecting an estimated 10 percent of adults. That's no surprise when you consider that folate is abundant in the foods that get the least attention in the typical American diet—vegetables.

Most of the publicity about folate deficiency concerns the risk of birth defects in babies born to vitamin-deficient mothers. Folate deficiency, however, is associated with another health problem—cancer. Studies show that people with low blood levels of dietary folate run a higher risk for some types of cancer. Conversely, studies show that people with high levels of dietary folate in their blood are protected from certain cancers.

When it comes to folate and cancer, however, there appears to be an issue of *quality*. You see, folic acid, the supplemental form of this important B vitamin, is not always an adequate stand-in for the real thing. But when it comes to cancer prevention, one thing is crystal clear. You don't want to ignore folate.

Why Folate Is Important

Folate is an essential cancer fighter due to the role it plays in cell life. Folate is responsible for creating red blood cells. It is also required for cell division. Folate, along with vitamin B_{12}, is essential to the synthesis of RNA and DNA, the architects of every cell in the body. Damaged DNA is the beginning of the long process that eventually leads to cell mutation and tumor formation.

We don't require a lot of folate to make this happen; the daily value is only 50 micrograms, but for optimum health and cancer prevention we could stand to get a lot more. When things go wrong—when we get sick or injured or our health is compromised by such things as cigarettes and booze—our need for folate rises. Studies show that people who eat lots of folate-rich foods have a lower risk of **breast** and **pancreatic cancers**. One population-based study of 1,700 women in Shanghai, who were not drinkers or supplement takers, found that those who consumed the most folate-rich foods had a significantly reduced risk of breast cancer compared to those who consumed the least. Another study of 27,101 healthy male smokers found that high dietary levels—but not supplements—had a "significantly protective effect" against **prostate cancer**. In fact, one long-term study found that male smokers who took folic acid supplements for 10 years had a 10 percent greater risk of getting prostate cancer compared to only a 3 percent greater risk in male smokers who took a placebo.

The majority of the research on dietary folate, however, shows that it is most powerful in fighting back **colon cancer**. One study of 14,407 people that spanned 20 years found 249 micrograms of dietary folate a day—the equivalent of eating a healthy serving of beans—offered substantial protection against colon cancer in non-smoking men.

Eating folate-rich foods did not have the same impact on women, but a different study that involved folic acid *supplements* told a different story. The study, conducted in Europe, followed the rate of colorectal cancer among women who took folic acid supplements for 15 years. Women who took the supplements had a lower risk of colorectal cancer than women who did not.

European researchers also found that folic acid supplements had protective effects against **pharyngeal** and **oral cavity cancers**. And one 10-year study of 35,023 women between the ages of 50 ad 76 found that taking folic acid supplements reduced the risk of **breast cancer**.

How Much to Take

Folate and folic acid supplements are water soluble, meaning they do not build up in fatty tissue, so they are not toxic. Researchers, however, fall short of recommending folic acid supplementation for the general public as a hedge against cancer. However, they do recommend supplements for high-risk individuals, even if they have normal blood levels of folate. The recommended dosage for optimum health is 400 micrograms a day.

Whether you take supplements or not, you should still make sure that you eat plenty of folate foods. Good sources of folate include liver, legumes, green leafy vegetables, citrus fruit, and juices. Breads, cereals, and grain products also are fortified with folate.

Folate can be lost from foods during preparation, cooking and storage. These strategies will help preserve the folate in the food you eat:

- Eat vegetables raw whenever possible.
- Store folate foods in the refrigerator.
- Steam, boil or simmer in the minimal amount of water.

GINSENG

It's called American but its origin is in Asia, where it has been used for centuries as a healing tonic for a host of ailments. These days ginseng is helping improve quality of life and increase the survival rate of people with cancer. It is also gaining attention as a potentially powerful cancer fighter.

Ginseng owes its healing powers to several immune-boosting chemicals called ginsenosides. Though these compounds are still somewhat of a mystery, Korean scientists have seen them fight tumors in both human and animal studies on a variety of levels. After analyzing data from studies spanning 15 years, the researchers believe ginseng has the ability to help halt cancer cell proliferation and cause cell death at several different sites. Though they say more study is warranted, the researchers concluded that "the intake of ginseng may reduce the risk of several types of cancer."

The ginsenosides in ginseng are best known for having both stimulating and inhibiting effects on the central nervous system. This is the action that most comes into play for patients with cancer. When the major Shanghai Breast Cancer Study began back in the 1980s, 27 percent of the women reported that they had been regular users of ginseng since before their cancer diagnosis. Years late, these women proved to have a significantly increased survival rate.

Ginseng proved to be a welcome dietary addition even to the women who started taking it after being diagnosed with cancer. Of the 1,455 patients enrolled in the study, ginseng users showed a significant increase in quality of life that only improved with cumulative use.

Deciphering Ginseng

There are several different types of ginseng but American and Asian are the best known, and best used. Both Asian ginseng *(Panx ginseng)* and American ginseng *(Panax quinquefolius)* were used in the Shanghai study.

The women in the Shanghai Breast Cancer Study who experienced positive results took either Asian or American ginseng, though the researchers considered American to be the most effective.

Siberian ginseng *(Eleutherococcus senticosus)* is another type of ginseng you might come across, but it is not true ginseng.

Look for extract of American or Asian ginseng standardized to 4 percent ginsenosides. Recommended dosage is 100 to 200 milligrams a day.

GRAPE SEED EXTRACT

For decades health food activists have been extolling the virtues of grape seed extract, and we are now starting to see what all the fuss is about. These days activists can chant *Take grape seed—stop cancer.*

Grape seed extract is a super-saturated source of anthocyanins, antioxidants that are found in the skin of grapes and certain other fruit. During the last several years, scientists have found just what these substances can do beneath the skin. Anthocyanins and other polyphenols in the extract have been shown to arrest cancerous cells in an impressive list of enemy targets—**breast**, **colorectal**, **lung**, **prostate**, **skin**, and **stomach cancers**.

In 2009, researchers at the University of Kentucky elevated grape seed extract to a new level. They gave the extract to lab rats injected with **leukemia** cells. It was impressive enough that the extract forced *76 percent* of the cells into remission, but what really amazed the researchers was that it did it *within hours*.

"These results could have implications for the incorporation of agents such as grape seed extract into prevention or treatment of hematological [blood cell] malignancies and possibly other cancers," said the study's lead author, Xianglin Shi, Ph.D.

The Kentucky researchers also figured out how grape seed extract does the job—something that had eluded researchers in previous studies. It appears that the extract can sniff out and "wake up" a specific protein called JNK that prompts damaged cells to self-destruct.

Studies show that grape seed extract may also hold promise for people undergoing cancer treatment by preventing liver cell damage caused by chemotherapy medications.

How Much to Take

Grape seed extract is generally sold in capsule form at varying doses. Experts recommend taking from 50 to 100 milligrams a day. Side effects are considered minor and include dizziness and nausea.

GREEN TEA EXTRACT

Most Americans don't drink a lot of tea, especially green tea, yet drinking 30 to 40 ounces a day of green tea—the amount commonly consumed daily in China and Japan—has been found to help prevent cancer. You can get the same effect without ever putting a teacup to your lips by taking green tea extract.

Green tea extract offers a concentrated dose of epigallocatechin gallate (EGCG), a compound well-known for its cancer-preventive properties. In studies, healthy people took 15 tablets (2.5 grams) of green tea extract a day for six months without any adverse side effects—the equivalent of drinking 40 ounces of the tea. In trials with lung cancer patients, doctors found the maximum tolerated dosage is 3 grams a day.

Most recently, researchers at Mayo Clinic found that not only are large doses of green tea extract tolerable, but EGCG, the active ingredient in green tea, helped reduce lymphocyte count in patients with a common and incurable type of **leukemia**.

"We found not only that patients tolerated the green tea extract at very high doses, but that many of them saw regression to some degree of their chronic lymphocytic leukemia," says Tait Shanafelt, M.D., Mayo Clinic hematologist and lead author of the study. "The majority of individuals who entered the study with enlarged lymph nodes saw a fifty percent or greater decline in their lymph node size."

How Much to Take

If you can't drink green tea all day every day like Asians do, you can opt for the extract. To get an anti-cancer effect, the recommended dosage is 2.5 grams, about 15 tablets. Even though studies show high doses of green tea extract are well tolerated, you could experience side effects. They include nausea, bloating, gas, heartburn, diarrhea, and vomiting.

LUTEIN

We hear a lot about beta-carotene—by far the best-known of a class of nutrients called carotenoids. But when it comes to the body's ability to absorb carotenoids, lutein leaves beta-carotene in the dust.

This has important implications in an anti-cancer diet because lutein, well known as the nutrient that helps prevent macular degeneration, plays an important role in **colon cancer**.

Scientists proved the power of lutein when they put 54 volunteers on a four-week diet rich in carotenoids. One group of 22 ate a high-vegetable daily diet consisting of 17.1 ounces of vegetables rich in both beta carotene and lutein. Another group of 22 ate a low-vegetable diet consisting of 4.5 ounces of the same vegetables. A third group of 10 people ate a low-vegetable diet supplemented with 6 milligrams of beta carotene and 9 milligrams of lutein. At the end of the four weeks, blood was taken from the volunteers to test nutrient levels. Vitamin C levels were significantly higher in those on the high-vegetable diet—no surprise there. But what did surprise researchers was that lutein levels were four times higher than beta-carotene levels—14 percent for beta-carotene and 67 percent for lutein!

In another experiment, researchers from the University of Utah Medical School in Salt Lake City measured the ability of three different carotinoids—beta carotene, lycopene and lutein—to reduce the risk of colon cancer. The study included 1,993 people diagnosed with colon cancer and 2,410 who were cancer-free. They found that those who ate the most foods high in lutein had a lower risk of the disease than people who ate foods low in lutein. More interestingly, lutein was the only carotenoid that proved to show any beneficial effect, especially among younger people.

They reported that the lycopene and beta carotene were "unremarkable" when it came to reducing the risk of colon cancer.

Lutein was also found to offer cancer protection to smokers.

The bottom line: Keep lutein on your radar when selecting vegetables, especially if you're at risk for colon cancer.

CAUTION: One study found that taking lutein may increase the risk of lung cancer in smokers.

Getting More Lutein in Your Diet

The best way to get lutein is through diet. Lutein can be found in many fruits and vegetables. The people who benefited from lutein in the Utah study reported that they ate these fruits and vegetables:

- Broccoli
- Carrots
- Celery
- Greens
- Lettuce
- Oranges
- Orange juice
- Spinach
- Tomatoes

Other lutein-rich foods include:

- Cabbage
- Green beans
- Kale
- Mangoes
- Papaya
- Peaches

If you don't get enough of these vegetables and fruits in your diet or you are at risk for colorectal cancer, you might want to consider a supplement. Look for lutein supplements containing zeatanthin. The recommended dosage is 10 milligrams daily. There are no known side effects at this dosage.

LYCOPENE

Some people think of tomatoes as a bottle of ketchup. Some researchers think of tomatoes as a bottle of lycopene.

Lycopene has been a nutrient of keen scientific interest ever since researchers observed that Mediterraneans, who eat a diet rich in fruits and vegetables, have one of the lowest rates of cancer in the world. Men in the Mediterranean region enjoy a particularly low rate of prostate cancer.

Lycopene is the richest source of a well-known class of cancer-fighting nutrients called carotenoids, which are abundant in tomatoes, a staple of the Mediterranean diet. Tomatoes and tomato products are the richest sources of lycopene, which is what led researchers to put one (lycopene) and one (tomatoes) together to see if they added up to a low rate of **prostate cancer**. It turns out that lycopene was found to not only protect against prostate cancer, but other cancers as well, including **bladder**, **breast**, **cervix**, **colorectal**, **esophageal**, and **ovarian cancers**.

Studies, however, have not been consistent. For example, one large-scale analysis of all the studies involving lycopene supplementation and cancer found that lycopene appeared to offer some protection against all cancers *except* for one—prostate. Other research reveals there may be an explanation for the inconsistent results. Lycopene, it appears, works harder when it gets help from other nutrients. In one study, for example, 500 Chinese men were divided into three groups. One group took lycopene supplements daily for several months. Another group drank green tea daily, and the third group took lycopene *and* drank green tea. Researchers found a reduced risk of prostate cancer in all three groups, but the men who took lycopene and drank green tea had the lowest risk of all.

Another study tested the power of supplemental lycopene and genistein, an isoflavone found in soy, on 71 men diagnosed with prostate cancer who had had three consecutive elevated readings on the PSA (prostate-specific antigen) test, a marker for possible cancer activity.

The patients were randomly selected to take a 15 milligram capsule of lycopene, or lycopene plus 40 milligrams of genistein, twice daily for six months. Both groups experienced a drop in PSA, but the lycopene and genistein proved to have the greater effect. Another study involving soy found progression of prostate cancer slowed down in men who took lycopene supplements and followed a low-fat vegan diet that included soy.

What This Means to You

It may take a genie in a bottle to reveal exactly how important lycopene supplements are to a cancer-protection program, but most experts agree that it is important to get the nutrient in the diet.

Tomatoes and tomato products by far are the richest source of lycopene. You'll find measurably more lycopene in a can of tomato sauce than a fresh tomato because lycopene activity increases with cooking. Other good sources of lycopene include:

- Asparagus
- Grapefruit
- Papaya
- Sweet red pepper
- Watermelon

If these foods are generally not on your active-eating list, you might want to consider a lycopene supplement. The recommended dosage is 15 milligrams a day.

MILK THISTLE

People with an alcohol capacity bigger than what's good for them might want to consider taking the herb milk thistle.

Milk thistle is an ancient "liver tonic" that modern doctors are finding may be beneficial for people at risk for **liver cancer**. Milk thistle's liver-protecting ability comes from silymarin, an antioxidant that is extracted from the seeds of the herb. Silymarin contains four compounds, the most active of which is silybin. Studies show that silymarin and silybin help protect the liver by blocking toxins from entering cells or by moving toxins out before trouble begins.

In one study of 170 patients with cirrhosis of the liver, including 46 alcoholics, half the people were treated with a special preparation containing 70 to 80 percent silymarin and the other half was given a placebo. After three years of treatment, those receiving the silymarin had a lower mortality rate than those who took a placebo. The alcoholics experienced the greatest benefit. Cirrhosis is a leading cause of liver cancer.

Several other studies found that people with chronic liver disease showed improvement after taking milk thistle for anywhere from four weeks to six months.

Laboratory and animal studies are finding that milk thistle may help prevent and treat a variety of cancers, including **bladder**, **colon**, **tongue**, **skin**, and **small intestine cancers**. Laboratory studies show that it may increase the effectiveness of chemotherapy drugs and make them less toxic.

How Much to Take
Milk thistle can be purchased as tablets or capsules. Look for milk thistle standardized to 80 percent silymarin. The recommended dosage ranges from 150 to 175 milligrams three times a day.

Milk thistle is generally considered safe and has no known side effects at the recommended dose.

PECTIN
If you need more fiber in your diet, you can conquer two problems with one swallow of a pectin supplement.

Pectin is a soluble fiber present in many plants but it is concentrated in the peel and pulp of apples, pears, and citrus fruit. Modified citrus pectin (MCP) is an altered form that is more absorbable than the natural pectin in fruit. Pectin is important to health because it possesses strong anti-cancer properties. However, it is proving to be especially important to cancer patients because laboratory and animal studies indicate it can help stop tumors from growing and spreading.

In one study, 10 men with **prostate cancer** received six capsules of MCP three times a day. After one year, there was a significant reduction in their PSA (prostate-specific antigen), the test used to detect possible cancer. Three of the men suffered mild side effects (abdominal cramps and diarrhea) from the dosage and had to drop

ASPIRIN: TO TAKE IT OR NOT IS STILL THE QUESTION

The verdict is in. Taking an aspirin a day can help prevent cancer. Although all doctors aren't ready to endorse it as an across-the-board strategy, most feel taking an aspirin a day to prevent cancer is probably a good idea, especially among younger people.

Aspirin blocks the effects of COX-2 enzymes, inflammatory proteins often found in high levels in people with cancer.

Several studies show that taking an aspirin a day, or another over-the-counter non-steroidal anti-inflammatory drug (NSAID), such as ibuprofen, can help prevent or at least delay **colorectal** and **prostate cancers** and possibly some others. Studies over the years show aspirin reduces the risk of benign tumors and prevents, at least in part, tumor growth. One study found that those who took an aspirin a day for at least 10 years lowered the risk of getting colorectal cancer later in life. Another study found that cancer patients taking aspirin had a lower death rate than those who didn't take aspirin.

A major analysis of 38 studies involving 2.7 million women showed that women who took aspirin had a 13 percent lower risk of breast cancer than those who didn't take aspirin. Women who took ibuprofen had a 21 percent reduced risk.

A study involving 29,000 men found that a daily aspirin reduced the risk of cancer by 14 percent. In men who reported taking two or more NSAIDs a day, the risk was even lower.

Continued

> Still, the researchers fell short of recommending a daily aspirin to prevent cancer. Aspirin can cause side effects, such as stomach ulcers and gastrointestinal bleeding. These side effects are more common in people over age 60, which is also the age at which the risk of cancer goes up.

out of the study, but the symptoms disappeared after they stopped taking the supplements.

Animal studies have found similar results with **melanoma**, **breast**, and **colon cancers**. One study showed that MCP helped prevent colon cancer from spreading to the liver, which is a risk associated with cancer surgery. In China, researchers exposed 75 mice to a medical state simulating metastatic post-operative cancer. They divided the mice into four groups that received no, low, medium or high doses of MCP. At three weeks, the no-dosage mice stomachs were bulging with new tumors. Other mice got metastatic disease as well, but their rate correlated with the amount of MCP they received. The higher the dosage, the lower the risk. The high-dose mice experienced significantly fewer metastatic tumors than the low-dose mice.

How Much to Take

Modified citrus pectin comes as both a powder and supplement. The recommended dosage for the powder is 1 teaspoon (5 grams) mixed with a large glass of water or juice three times a day. The recommended dosage for the capsules is 800 milligrams three times a day.

Side effects are rare, but large dosages could result in stomach upset.

RESVERATROL

The jury may still be out on whether drinking wine plays an important role in preventing cancer, but one thing is certain. Resveratrol, the active ingredient that gets all the credit for making wine a health food, is one mighty powerful cancer fighter.

When Columbia University researchers went in "search for novel and effective cancer chemopreventive agents," they hit the jackpot when they got to R for resveratrol. Here's what they found:

Brain cancer. Mice with brain tumors were given resveratrol daily for 28 days. Researchers found that the supplement suppressed tumor growth, resulting in a 70 percent increase in long-term survival.

Breast cancer. Alcohol promotes estrogen production, which is why drinking raises the risk for breast cancer. (Excessive estrogen raises the risk.) However, resveratrol supplements helped prevent breast cancer, at least in rats. When rats were injected with breast cancer cells, resveratrol delayed the development of tumors. It also reduced the ability of the cancer to metastasize.

Colorectal cancer. In one study, mice that had been implanted with colorectal cancer cells were given resveratrol diluted in water for seven weeks. The resveratrol helped prevent cancer in three ways. It reduced tumor formation in the small intestines, prevented tumors from developing in the colon, and prevented colon cancer genes from expressing. Tumor formation in the small intestines was reduced 70 percent.

Esophageal cancer. Resveratrol suppressed both the number and size of tumors in rats exposed to polyaromatic hydrocarbons, known carcinogens in cigarettes associated with esophageal cancer.

Fibrosarcoma. Resveratrol supplements inhibited

the formation and growth of cells that lead to this cancer of connective tissue.

Leukemia. A number of laboratory studies found that resveratrol induced tumor cell death leading to certain types of blood cancer.

Liver cancer. Several rat studies found that resveratrol's antioxidant activity can protect the liver from cancer in several ways. In one study, rats were given supplemental resveratrol for 10 days. At the end of the experiment, cancer progression had stopped in rats with both early- and late-stage disease. Another study found resveratrol protected the liver by neutralizing toxic substances.

Lung cancer. Resveratrol inhibited several carcinogens in cigarettes from metabolizing in test tube studies. It also reduced the number of lung tumors by 42 percent, the size of the tumors by 44 percent, and the ability of the tumors to metastasize by 56 percent.

Non-malignant melanoma. When resveratrol was applied topically to the skin of hairless mice that spent too much time (on purpose) in the sun, researchers found it "significantly inhibited" the toxic effects of harmful UVB rays. They also found that one single application of resveratrol on hairless mouse skin 30 minutes before sunbathing inhibited cancerous lesions. Applying it either before or after didn't seem to make a difference. In both instances, resveratrol prevented tumors from forming and inhibited precancerous lesions from getting worse.

The same can't be said for all skin cancers, however. When mice were given mouse-size supplements equivalent to the human dose of 20 milligrams a day, it showed no effect on the prevention of malignant melanoma, the most deadly form of the disease.

Pancreatic cancer. Laboratory studies found that

resveratrol inhibited proliferation of human pancreatic cancer cells, although the same results were not found in hamsters inoculated with tumor cells.

Stomach cancer. Resveratrol has the ability to inhibit *H. pylori*, the bacterium that causes ulcers and can lead to stomach cancer.

Prostate cancer. Several animal studies found that resveratrol fights prostate cancer on a variety of levels in both initial and advanced stages.

How Much to Take

Virtually all the studies on resveratrol supplements to date have been conducted on animals, so it still remains to be seen how effective it will be when used in human trials. However, supplements are the only way to get this protection without drinking wine. Plus, supplements offer what you can't get from drinking a glass or two of wine a day—a big infusion of resveratrol. You would have to drink *thousands* of glasses of wine to get the amount of resveratrol found in one supplement tablet.

Resveratrol is rare in food and red wine is the most abundant dietary source. It is also present in peanuts and berries.

The recommended dosage is 20 milligrams a day. Resveratrol is generally considered safe at this dosage. Side effects are rare and can include anemia, anxiety, diarrhea, and over-thinning of the blood.

ROSEMARY EXTRACT

To protect you and your family's health at barbecue time, keep a bottle of rosemary extract close to the grill. Researchers at Kansas State University found that applying rosemary extract to hamburgers can break the build-up of cancer-causing substances that accumulate when they are cooked at high temperatures. Extract is also an easy substitute if you don't have the herb on hand or don't care for its taste, especially in hambugers.

Rosemary, a member of the mint family and a popular herb, gets its cancer-protective action from special phenolic compounds, including rosmarinic acid, that prevent the formation of heterocyclic amines (HCAs) from building up on meat, poultry and fish grilled at a temperature higher than 352°F. HCAs have been associated with **stomach**, **colon**, and **pancreatic cancers**.

Using rosemary extract will allow you to cook at the temperature you want without altering the taste of the food, says J. Scott Smith, KSU science professor. Just put a few drops on the surface of the meat before grilling.

CAUTION: Make sure you buy edible rosemary extract, which you can find online or at health food stores Do not confuse it with rosemary (rosmarinic) aromatherapy oil.

SELENIUM
This trace mineral, which we get from food grown in selenium-rich soil, appears to play an important role in cancer prevention.

This first came to light when scientists noticed that selenium deficiency appeared to raise the risk of getting certain cancers. In parts of the world where selenium content in soil is low, rates of certain cancers are high. This is especially true among nations with selenium-poor soil that are dependent solely on locally grown foods. In areas where soil is rich in selenium, cancer rates are low. In Greece, for example, where the soil is rich in selenium, men enjoy the lowest rates of prostate cancer in the world.

Research over the last several decades indicates that

selenium targets specific cancers. U.S. researchers found that people who have a precancerous condition known as Barrett's esophagus *and* low selenium levels had double the risk of **esophageal cancer**. When Canadian researchers analyzed the results of 16 **prostate cancer** studies, they found that men who took selenium supplements had a 28 percent reduced risk of the cancer. In another study, they found that men with high blood levels of selenium had a 39 percent lower risk of the disease.

Researchers at the University of Arizona's Arizona Cancer Center analyzed several studies that looked at selenium levels and **colorectal cancer** and found that those with the highest blood levels of the nutrient had a 34 percent lower risk of developing the disease. In ex-smokers at increased risk for **bladder cancer**, selenium supplements reduced their risk in half (along with kicking the habit).

Selenium contains special antioxidants called selenoproteins that attack cancer cells by cutting off their blood supply, which essentially causes them to suffocate and die. A 2009 study at the University of Texas M.D. Anderson Cancer Center in Houston found selenium might work even better when combined with another powerful antioxidant, vitamin E. In their experiment, the Anderson researchers found that 200 micrograms of selenium and 400 I.U. of vitamin E daily not only had the ability to suppress tumors, but also stopped cancer genes from expressing.

How Much to Take

While most Americans are not deficient in selenium, it is hard to figure how much selenium you are getting from food because mineral content is soil-dependent. The only super-rich source of selenium is Brazil nuts.

Just 1 ounce provides more than 10 times the daily value.

The daily value for selenium is 55 micrograms but the doses used in research to get cancer-fighting results are much higher. One study of 1,300 Americans found that 200 micrograms daily of supplemental selenium reduced overall cancer rates by 41 percent after 10 years.

Selenium is toxic at high rates. The upper safe level of supplemental selenium is considered to be 400 micrograms.

VITAMIN C

Ever since the late Nobel laureate Linus Pauling suggested that taking large vitamin C supplements can help prevent cancer, this common and harmless nutrient has been cast in controversy.

There is no doubt that vitamin C has an iron arm when it flexes its antioxidant muscle in a match with cancer. Numerous human studies show that dietary vitamin C and vitamin C supplements can help reduce the risk of cancer. Vitamin C has also been used to treat certain cancers. The roster includes **cervical**, **esophageal**, **lung**, **pancreatic**, **pharyngeal**, **oral cavity**, and **stomach cancers**. Most of the studies, however, suggest that it takes therapeutically large dosages—up to several grams—to get the effect. Considering that the average daily requirement to sustain good health is 60 to 90 milligrams, that's a whole lot of vitamin C.

For every study that says taking vitamin C supplements can help prevent cancer, there's another that says it is a waste of money. However, an international panel of cancer experts concluded in 2003 that vitamin C is important in combating cancer.

Vitamin C helps guard against cancer in a variety of ways. It stimulates the immune system, and blocks the activation of tumor cells. It also can fight the toxic effects of carcinogens in cigarettes and air pollution. The international committee that gave vitamin C its blessing says it can do all these things and more because it is simply one mighty antioxidant.

"Because tumor promotion is closely linked to oxidative and inflammatory processes and because it is a relatively long and reversible process, antioxidant-rich whole foods such as fruit, vegetables, and grains can efficiently reverse and suppress the carcinogenic process," the group reported in the *American Journal of Clinical Nutrition.* "Thus, the consumption of 5 servings of fruit and vegetables containing 200–280 mg vitamin C could be still recommended, although further research is needed to establish whether vitamin C supplementation beyond normal dietary intake is beneficial."

How Much to Take

So, how much vitamin C should you take to help guard against cancer? British researchers went looking for the answer to this question when they put individuals on vitamin C supplements up to dosages of 500 milligrams a day for six weeks. They found that supplements provided cell protection, but only at levels of 100 to 200 milligrams a day.

Vitamin C is generally considered safe, though there can be side effects at high levels. They include nausea, vomiting, diarrhea, and headache. Even at doses as small as 100 milligrams, you may have to build up your tolerance to avoid side effects. You can minimize any side-effects by spreading out intake throughout the day.

Vitamin C is readily available in fruits and vegetables. Some of the best sources include:

- Bell peppers
- Broccoli
- Brussels sprouts
- Guava
- Kale
- Kiwi
- Mangoes
- Oranges
- Sweet potatoes
- Tomato juice

VITAMIN D

Three out of four Americans don't get enough vitamin D, which may be raising their risk for certain kinds of cancers.

At one time, vitamin D deficiency was only associated with rickets in children and bone loss in adults. However, studies over the last several years have found that vitamin D is important protection against cancer. Several studies found that taking 1,000 IU of vitamin D, known as the sunshine vitamin, can reduce the risk of **breast**, **colon**, **prostate**, **ovarian**, and **skin cancers** by up to 50 percent.

"The high prevalence of vitamin D deficiency, combined with the discovery of increased risks of certain types of cancer in those who are deficient, suggest that vitamin D deficiency may account for several thousand premature deaths from colon, breast, ovarian, and other cancers annually," says Cedric F. Garland, a researcher and cancer specialist at Moores Cancer Center at the University of California in San Diego. Researchers believe Vitamin D helps block certain cancer cells from forming and dividing.

The high rate of vitamin D deficiency reported in

2009 was attributed primarily to overzealous use of sunscreen and insufficient outdoor activity. Those most at risk are believed to be people who live in the Northeast and those with a lot of melanin in the skin, a pigment that helps protect against ultraviolet rays of the sun. Garland noted that pigmentation could be one of the reasons African Americans are at higher risk for some cancers. The sun is the major source of vitamin D. Fortified milk is the major food source of vitamin D.

How Much to Take

The preponderance of evidence linking vitamin D deficiency to cancer and other health risks has encouraged many officials to call for an increase in the minimum daily value, which is currently 200 IU up to age 50, 400 IU for ages 51 to 79, and 600 IU for age 71 and older. Other than the sun, there are no excellent sources of the vitamin, as a glass of milk only has 100 IU of vitamin D.

The recommended dosage for cancer prevention is 1,000 IU daily.

VITAMIN E

Vitamin E is a hard-working antioxidant that isn't all that easy to get from food, mostly because it is found in oils. Vitamin E is important, however, and plays a central role in cancer prevention, because it helps protect against the cell damage that begins the corrosive process that ends up as cancer.

Vitamin E has a direct link to cancer prevention. It has been found to block the formation of nitrosamines, carcinogens found in tobacco, and nitrites, a food additive that has been linked to cancer. It's also an important immune-enhancing nutrient.

The benefits of vitamin E *supplementation* are somewhat muddled because results of numerous studies conducted over the last two decades have been contradictory. Some of the most promising results, however, have been found for **breast** and **prostate cancers**.

The ongoing Nurses' Health Study involving 83,234 women found that vitamin E offered a significant 43 percent reduction in the risk of **breast cancer** in premenopausal women with a family history of the disease, but only a 16 percent reduction in risk among other women. The researchers concluded vitamin E supplements may be protective only against genetically caused breast cancer.

Vitamin E comes in many forms—standard vitamins are sold as alpha-tocopherol—and it is possible that other forms of the vitamin are more protective against cancer in people with specific risk factors. Analysis conducted by researchers at Wake Forest University School of Medicine found that another form of vitamin E—tocotrienols—not only showed the most protection against breast cancer, but also helped stop the cancer from spreading.

One long-term study of 29,361 male smokers in Finland did not find that vitamin E supplementation reduced the risk of lung cancer, but it did find that it helped protect them from prostate cancer. After eight years, the researchers found that vitamin E reduced the risk of prostate cancer by 32 percent. It also reduced the risk of dying from it by 41 percent. Researchers at the National Institutes of Health noted, however, that there are no statistics to prove that vitamin E's protective effects extend to non-smokers.

Animal studies have found that vitamin E supplements reduced the risk of dying from **bladder cancer**

and may help prevent **colon cancer** and **melanoma**.
Whether the same effects can be found in humans is
yet to be seen.

There is no question, however, that vitamin E plays
a role in cancer prevention. Italian doctors who did a
mega-analysis of European studies found that people
who eat foods high in vitamin E had a reduced risk of
several kinds of cancer, including **breast**, **esophageal**,
gallbladder, **pharyngeal**, and **oral cavity cancers**.

What This Means to You

It appears the best way to approach vitamin E is to increase it in your diet. Wheat germ and vegetable oils are
the richest sources. You can also find it in these foods:

- Apples
- Blackberries
- Black currants
- Mango
- Nuts
- Salad dressings
- Sunflower seeds
- Whole grains

If you don't consume these foods frequently, you
might want to consider a vitamin E supplement. Vitamin E as alpha-tocopherol is the most popular and
commonly sold supplement. It comes as a soft gel capsule. The recommended dosage is 400 IU. You can also
get the vitamin as tocotrienols plus E complex, which
you should take according to package directions. For
the best vitamin E absorption, take it with a meal containing some fat, such as olive oil or fish oil.

The vitamin is generally considered safe in recommended dosages. Side effects that indicate you may be getting too much include fatigue, upset stomach, diarrhea, gas, headache, and blurred vision.

CAUTION: Several studies have suggested that vitamin E supplementation may be associated with increased risk of **cervical**, **colorectal**, and **lung cancers**.

CHAPTER 6

How to Create an Anti-cancer Lifestyle

By arming your diet with anti-cancer foods and fortifying your immune defense with anti-cancer supplements, you are making a major effort in helping to protect yourself against cancer. But this is only part of an all-out cancer-prevention strategy. You also need to examine and, if necessary, adjust your lifestyle.

Cancer researchers believe that what we eat *and* how we choose to live our lives go hand in hand when it comes to taking action to help stop cancer. The measures that offer you the best defense against cancer are:

- Getting all recommended cancer screenings at the recommended age and on time.
- Eating a diet rich in cancer-fighting foods—a minimum of four to five servings, or 14 ounces, a day of fruits and vegetables.
- Limiting red and processed meat consumption to 3 ounces or less a day.
- Taking immune-fortifying, cancer-fighting supplements.
- Avoiding cigarettes and secondhand smoke.
- Protecting yourself against the sun.

- Living an active lifestyle that includes two and a half hours a week of moderately intense exercise.
- Avoiding hard liquor, and drinking wine or beer in moderation.
- Minimizing your exposure to pollution and radiation, if and when possible.
- Testing your home for radon and taking steps to decrease levels in your home, if necessary.
- Recognizing your personal cancer risk factors and taking appropriate action to minimize them.

Living an anti-cancer lifestyle is no guarantee that you will avoid cancer, but it can help reduce your odds. And should you get cancer, having a history of healthy lifestyle practices will help increase your chances of survival. Researchers at the University of Michigan Comprehensive Cancer Center investigated the lifestyle habits of 504 cancer patients at diagnosis and followed them for several years to see how lifestyle impacted their survival odds. They found that smoking, problem drinking, a poor diet, lack of sleep, and little exercise were associated with the worst odds for survival.

Reducing the risk for cancer is a lifestyle, one that includes eating important cancer-fighting foods and trying to keep your environment safe. There is no such thing as a toxic-free environment but there are things you can do to minimize your exposure to a majority of cancer-causing threats. These are the major lifestyle practices that should be getting your attention.

IF YOU SMOKE, QUIT

If you smoke and want to quit, you are far from alone. An estimated 1.3 billion people worldwide smoke and 70 percent of them say they would like to kick the habit. If you are among them, you know it's a big leap from desire to action, and an even bigger leap from action to success.

But don't give up trying, because there are plenty of reasons for you to shoot for success. Most people want to quit smoking for personal reasons—family, job, health, the desire to breathe in a lungful of clean fresh air. They all mean more than the addictive pleasure that comes from smoking a cigarette.

Addictions are hard to break and, unfortunately, smoking is one of the toughest, but here's a fact that should help your motivation: Your risk of getting cancer (and smoking can lead to 13 different types) *starts to go down the moment you put out your last cigarette.*

Even if you're already in middle age with 20 or 30 years of smoking behind you, you can still win back many of the years you might have lost to smoking. Those who never smoked may have better odds of not getting a smoking-related cancer than former smokers, but former smokers are far better off than current smokers.

There are many programs and products available to help you stop smoking, including the one many former smokers found effective—going cold turkey.

Out of all the resources available to help beat the tobacco habit, studies have found the three listed on the opposite page have the best odds for success.

Keep in mind that pharmaceuticals, whether prescription or over the counter, carry side effects and may not be right for your health status. If you want to go the drug route, discuss the options with your doctor first.

Like dieting, quitting smoking often can be easier when done in the company of others in the same boat or with the kind encouragement of a supporter. Studies have found the interventions on page 202 to be most effective.

Program	How It Is Sold	How It Works	Duration	Success Rate
Vareninicline	Prescription	Reduces cravings and decreases pleasurable effects of cigarettes	12 weeks. If successful, can be continued for another 12 weeks to prevent recurrence	Threefold compared to placebo
Bupropion (Wellbutrin, Zycam)	Prescription	Antidepressant that has been found to decrease the severity of cravings and withdrawal symptoms	8 weeks. If successful, can be taken for up to a year to prevent recurrence	Twofold compared to placebo
Nicotene replacement therapy, sold as patch, gum, inhaler or lozenge	Over the counter	Helps relieve withdrawal symptoms	8–12 weeks. If successful, can be taken for up to a year to prevent recurrence	One-and-a-half- to twofold compared to placebo

Intervention	How It Works
One-on-one counseling	This is done with a health-care professional other than current providers. Short-term can be just as effective as long-term.
Social support	This focuses on adapting to a smoke-free environment, such as in the home or workplace. A counselor may have to meet with family, friends, and coworkers in out-of-the-ordinary situations.
Group counseling	These forums offer advice on behavioral techniques for nicotine withdrawal and the benefit of sharing experiences with others in a like situation.
Telephone counseling	A trained supporter, either a health-care professional or former smoker, is at your service to offer support when needed or at a scheduled time.
Self-help materials	Videos, audios, websites, and printed materials are available to assist smokers on stop-smoking options and what to expect during withdrawal.

Don't Be a Switch Smoker

Trading in cigarettes for cigars or a pipe only trades one risk for another. Whether you inhale or not, the risk of cancer increases with the length of time you use tobacco, be it cigarettes, cigars or pipes. In fact, records show higher rates of **lung cancer** among people who switched from cigarettes to cigars or a pipe than in people who smoke cigars or a pipe exclusively.

The same holds true for chewing tobacco. One U.S. study found that men who switched from cigarettes to chewing tobacco had a death rate that was 2.6 times higher from **oral cancer** than those who gave up smoking entirely. Compared to men who never smoked, the risk of lung cancer among switchers increased five- to six-fold.

If You Don't Smoke, Help Others to Quit

Have loved ones who smoke? It appears that there is an effective way to nag them into quitting. The technique? Send them warning messages on their computers or cell phone about the health consequences of smoking.

Researchers found this to be an effective strategy quite by accident after trying it out on a volunteer group of young smokers from North Dakota University. The experiment was intended to explore ways of communicating smoking-related information, but was not targeted at trying to get them to quit. But that's not how it turned out.

Students were divided into two groups. One group was sent messages focused on hassles in life, such as stress and money. The other group received anti-smoking messages. These messages included reminders about how smoking causes wrinkles and yellow teeth, the impact of secondhand smoke on others, and how "93

percent of lung cancer patients die within five years."
The messages were sent eight times a day for one week
and six times a day during the next week. More than
half of the people getting the serious anti-smoking messages said they tried to quit during the intervention.
Only 19 percent in the other group reported that they
tried to quit.

The anti-smoking messages were the motivating factor that influenced them to quit. "Worry seems to be
part of what's important," said Danielle McCarthy, of
Rutgers University, who was involved in the study. The
bottom line: Warning messages create worry that can
nudge smokers into making the decision to quit.

Ban Smoke-Filled Rooms

Smokers know how hard it is to give up smoking—an
admirable feat that goes largely unrewarded if they
are constantly exposed to other people's smoke. There
is much debate over whether or not secondhand smoke
kills, but there is no question that it does harm. How
else is cotinine, a byproduct of nicotine, getting into
the bloodstream of non-smoking adults and children?

The good news is that smoking bans are working.
Three months after New York City implemented a
citywide smoking ban in July 2003, smoke-associated
symptoms among hospitality industry workers dropped
88 percent. Elsewhere, scientists are finding significant
reductions in the amount of nicotine residue in the
blood of non-smokers as a result of smoking bans in of-
fices, restaurants and public places. The bans are even
having a welcome, though not totally unexpected, side-
effect—smokers are cutting back.

Neverthleless, smoking bans are not everywhere, especially in the United States where they are mandated

by local or state legislation. Studies of non-smokers with lung cancer show that the most common exposure to secondhand smoke comes from three main sources: spouse, workplace, and social settings.

The Boston University School of Public Health did a study to identify the smokiest public places and came up with what it called "the 5 Bs": bars, bowling alleys, billiard halls, betting establishments, and bingo parlors. If there are no smoking bans in your community, these are the places you should try to avoid.

Get Proactive about Smoking Regulations

Secondhand smoke travels, so smoking bans are only as effective as they are widespread. On Feb. 27, 2005, the World Health Organization (WHO) declared war on tobacco, "reaffirming the right of all people to the highest standard of health." The goal is to curb and eventually eliminate tobacco use around the world. WHO is urging all countries to enforce legislation aimed at decreasing consumption, protecting non-smokers, and discouraging young people from starting. In addition to bans on smoking in public places, initiatives include public information campaigns, bans on tobacco advertising and promotion, and placing conspicuously large health warnings on cigarette packaging.

Some 30 countries, including Iceland, Ireland, England, and Scotland, have out-and-out banned smoking in all public places and workplaces nationwide, which gives non-smokers unprecedented protection from secondhand smoke. Ireland, by far, has the strictest regulations. Smoking is not allowed within a three-mile radius of any public area, indoors or outdoors, and violators can be jailed.

The United States, so far, has skirted a nationwide

ban. To date, only 15 states have bans on smoking in all public places, including restaurants and bars. Fifteen others have statewide bans with fewer limitations. Overall, the regulations protect only 50 percent of Americans, and only in varying degrees. There are many ways beyond smoking bans to help discourage smoking. Studies in industrial countries found that smoking dropped 2.5 to 3 percent with the initiation of a tax that raised the price of cigarettes 10 percent. One study in Europe found a 10 percent price hike resulted in a 5 to 7 percent drop in consumption.

Price hikes are discouraging young people from taking up the habit. A sophisticated analysis taken by a U.S. research firm showed that every $1 increase in a pack of cigarettes results in a 24 percent decline in smoking in one way or another, such as quitting, cutting back, stopping after experimenting with tobacco, or making the decision to never start.

You can help the dual goal to ban secondhand smoke and cut back on cigarette sales (and, thus, smoking) by supporting efforts and encouraging legislative action in your local community.

LIVE LEAN, STAY LEAN

When it comes to cancer odds, what you weigh may count even more than what you eat.

Researchers came to this assumption after studying the rate of obesity-related cancers among vegetarians around the world. They observed that people who maintained normal weight throughout life had an overall cancer risk that was even lower than in people whose diets largely depended on fruits and vegetables. This is a somewhat unsettling thought when you consider that overweight and obesity in the United States are rising to epidemic proportions. Cancer experts fear that as obesity rises, incidence of cancer will also rise. "In the coming decades, if there is no reversal in the currently observed trends, obesity and overweight will significantly contribute to further increases in cancer incidence," states the International Agency for Research on Cancer in *World Cancer Report 2008*.

Why BMI Is Important

Scientists determine overweight and obesity based on Body Mass Index (BMI). Ideal weight is considered a BMI between 20 and 23. Risk begins at a BMI of 25, the magic number that means you are overweight, and rises exponentially. A BMI of 30 or higher puts you in the obesity category.

The BMI does have some flaws in terms of what you see in the mirror. BMI is the same for men and women and it does not take into account bone structure or age. This means normal for a 5'5" man or woman, age 25 or 65, is somewhere between 114 and 150 pounds, and overweight doesn't count until you hit 150 pounds. So, be realistic when checking your BMI. A woman should aim for the lower end of this scale and a man can feel safe at the upper end. But, in the end, let the mirror be the judge. To see where you fit on the BMI scale, see the chart on page 209.

Another way scientists measure risk in relationship to overweight is by hip-to-waist ratio. Risk begins over a score of 0.8, which is considered normal. Finding your ratio involves elementary math. First, measure your waist just above the navel. Next, stand naked and wrap a measuring tape around your waist at the widest part. Then, divide your waist measurement by your hip measurement. For example: a 28-inch waist divided by 38-inch hips = 0.74.

Realistically, your ideal weight is a healthy weight that you can easily maintain without much effort. Though there is a theory that calorie restriction lowers the risk for certain diseases, there is no definitive proof that it is beneficial in preventing cancer, research shows.

Lose Weight Naturally

If you have a weight problem, eating the foods recommended in this book and exercising should help you gradually get to your ideal weight, as long as you do not take in more calories than you burn. Everyone burns calories at a different rate, depending on metabolic rate, physical activity, and body fat.

Here are some judicious guidelines to help you lose weight naturally:

Mind your fat. The same rules that apply for general health also apply for cancer prevention and weight loss. Get no more than 30 percent of your total daily calories from fat and keep your saturated fat intake below 10 percent of total calories.

Put a stopper on healthy oils. Even though healthy vegetable oils, such as olive and canola, are recommended in this book, they can add on the calories. A tablespoon of fat is still 100 percent fat and weighs in at 120 calories. You need no more than a tablespoon or two of either a day to get the anti-cancer effect.

Eat a little a lot. Many weight loss experts recommend eating five or six small meals instead of the three squares a day. Smaller meals help you lose and maintain weight because insulin levels stay normal and erratic insulin encourages fat storage.

Keep it natural. If it is processed, comes in a box, or contains sugar, refined flour, or trans fats, then it's not natural and will threaten your ability to lose weight.

BODY MASS INDEX			
	BMI 19–24.9	BMI 25–29.9	BMI 30 and above
Height (ft./in.)	Normal (lbs.)	Overweight (lbs.)	Obese (lbs.)
5'	97–127	128–157	158+
5'1"	100–131	132–163	164+
5'2"	104–135	136–168	169+
5'3"	107–140	141–174	175+
5'4"	110–144	145–179	180+
5'5"	114–149	150–185	186+
5'6"	118–154	155–191	192+
5'7"	121–158	159–197	198+
5'8"	125–163	164–202	203+
5'9"	128–168	169–208	209+
5'10"	132–173	174–215	216+
5'11"	136–178	179–221	222+
6'	140–183	184–227	228+
6'1"	144–174	182–219	227+
6'2"	148–186	194–225	233+
6'3"	152–192	200–232	240+

KEEP PHYSICALLY ACTIVE

There is overwhelming evidence that physical activity has a protective effect against cancer risk that improves as activity increases. There is also proof that a sedentary lifestyle contributes to the cause of some cancers.

For years, studies suggested that there is a link between exercise and risk of **breast cancer**, but the most powerful proof came in 2009 with the results of a 26-year study involving more than 14,000 women. The women were between the ages of 20 and 83 and cancer-free when the study began in 1973.

The study found that women who don't exercise or exercise very little are nearly three times more likely to die from breast cancer. The more exercise, the stronger the protection. The most fit women exercised at an intense rate for an average of five hours a week. "The results suggest a stronger protective effect than has been seen in most studies," noted Dr. Steve Blair, one of the researchers and a past president of the American College of Sports Medicine.

The researchers were even able to determine the minimum amount of exercise required to get a protective effect—two and a half hours a week of moderately intense exercise, including walking. The study also showed that effort can be accumulated in small 10-minute bouts.

Exercise is also important in reducing another risk—overweight. Older women who are overweight have a higher risk for **endometrial cancer**. One study of 109,621 women, ages 50 to 71, found that exercising five times a week helped reduce their risk.

An ambitious new study is adding considerable weight to the claim that exercise can lower the risk for **colorectal cancer**. Researchers at Washington University School of Medicine in St. Louis and Harvard University combined and analyzed several decades of data from past studies on how exercise affects risk. They found that men and women who exercised the most were 24 percent less likely to develop the disease than those who exercised the least.

"What's really compelling is that we see the association between exercise and lower colon cancer risk regardless of how physical activity was measured in the studies," said lead study author Dr. Kathleen Y. Wolin, a cancer prevention and control expert with the Siteman Cancer Center at Barnes-Jewish Hospital and Washington University. "That indicates that this is a robust association and gives all the more evidence that physical activity is truly protective against colon cancer."

The study found the protective effect included all types of physical activity, whether that activity was recreational, such as jogging, biking, or swimming, or job-related, such as walking, lifting, or digging. And it holds for both men and women. "There is an ever-growing body of evidence that the behavior choices we make affect our cancer risk," sais Wolin. "Physical activity is at the top of the list of ways that can reduce your risk of colon cancer."

To reduce your risk of cancer, the American Cancer Society recommends a minimum of 30 minutes of moderate exercise five or more times a week. And remember, the more active you are, the greater your protection against cancer will be.

Get Your Kids Moving, Too

Making physical activity a family activity is a must. At one time, parents could depend on school to get their kids on the move, but not anymore. Today, recess and physical education classes seem to be the exception rather than the rule.

On top of that, kids are less active once school is over. According to the latest statistics, 61.5 percent of children ages nine to 13 do not participate in any organized physical activity during nonschool hours.

It all points to a grim start for reducing the risk of life-threatening diseases, such as cancer. It's a well-established fact that underactive children become overweight adults. Over the past three decades, the proportion of overweight kids has doubled among two- to five-year-olds and tripled among six- to 19-year-olds. An estimated 14 percent of kids age two to five and 17.5 percent of kids ages six to 11 are considered overweight.

PRACTICE SAFE SUN

A tan is a twentieth-century fad that's fading away. At least that's what cancer experts are hoping. Not only is there no such thing as a healthy tan, there is no such thing as safe tanning, even if you avoid burning by dousing yourself in sunscreen.

Yes, even if you're the type who doesn't burn, you are vulnerable to skin cancer, especially basal cell and squamous cell carcinomas. Evidence shows that ultraviolet radiation can induce oxidative damage in cells at doses lower than required to produce a burn on the surface of the skin.

These are the two main rules of sun safety: If you're going to sunbathe, you need to protect your skin with sunscreen. And, if you're going to be in the sun for hours on end—playing volleyball or cruising on a boat, for instance—you need to wear more than sunscreen and a bathing suit.

How to Be Sunscreen-Sensible

As for sunscreen, it isn't going to do you much good if you don't use it properly, and many people don't. Here's what experts recommend:

- Use a sunscreen with a skin protective factor (SPF) of 15—no more. Not only is a higher SPF a waste of money, the chemicals in it tend to break down in the sun, so you are really only getting the same protection that you'd get from a 15 anyway.
- If you are so fair that you need an SPF of 30 or 50 to protect your skin, then your skin should not be exposed to the full sun at all. Wear a cover-up and a hat and sit under the protection of an umbrella or tree.
- Apply sunscreen heavily and only to parts of the body that will be exposed to the sun.
- Put the sunscreen on while you are still indoors, not when you're on the beach or by the pool.
- Limit your sun and beach activity time to a few hours and do so during the times when the sun is less powerful—before 10 a.m. and after 3 p.m.

It should go without saying that sunscreen is an absolute requirement for children, because sunburns in childhood are the greatest predictors of getting skin cancer as an adult. Also, sunscreen should not be put on babies less than six months old. In fact, the best practice is to keep all babies off the beach and out of the sun.

How to Be Sun Sensible

Some people can't avoid the sun. Boaters, fishermen, park workers, gardeners, tour guides, and lifeguards are among the many who spend all day in the sun. And there are others who simply won't avoid staying out in it, even if they can. Whether your exposure to the sun is for work or pleasure, a two-hour al fresco lunch or a four-hour walk in the park, follow these practices:

Cover up. Put sunscreen on all parts of the skin that will be exposed to the sun, even if it is only your face and hands. Wear long pants and long sleeves, if possible. You'll stay cool by choosing loose, natural fabrics. Dark colors are more protective than light colors.

Also, wear a wide-brimmed hat large enough to protect the scalp, ears, nose, and neck. Most importantly, protect your eyes by wearing sunglasses.

Seek shade often. Take shade breaks often, be it an awning, canopy, cove, or shade tree. People who are intentionally spending long hours in the sun should seek shade every half hour.

Stay dry. If you get wet, get into dry clothes as soon as possible. Wet clothes are less protective than dry clothes.

Beware of sun-sensitive foods. Certain foods and medicines are photosensitive, meaning even skin that doesn't burn will burn if exposed to the sun. Common offenders include citrus fruit and juices, celery, parsley, antibiotics, and antihistamines. In other words, drinking bloody Marys at the beach bar may not be a good idea.

Check out the UV Index. The Environmental Protection Agency (EPA) publishes a solar alert during the months when the sun is most harmful. The UV Index ranges from 1 to 10-plus. The EPA advises that you exercise caution in the sun when the UV Index exceeds 5 and to avoid it when it gets higher than an 8.

Cut your beach time in half. Here's the rule of thumb for recreating in coastal areas. Sand and water reflect the sun and double your skin's exposure to harmful UVB rays. If you can tolerate two hours sitting in the backyard, your safe time on the beach or water is one hour. Yes, even if you're wearing sunscreen.

BE SENSIBLE ABOUT DRINKING

An occasional drink, or even a drink every day, shouldn't raise your cancer risk, but what you choose to drink and when might help bring it down. If you're going to drink, the healthiest way to do so is to have a glass of wine with dinner.

One study examined the health risks among people who preferred either hard liquor, beer, or wine. All the people in the study were considered moderate drinkers, meaning they had no more than a drink or two a day. Wine drinkers proved to be the healthiest; the hard liquor drinkers had the most health complaints. Beer drinkers came in neutral.

Wine should be your drink of choice because it is abundant in nutrients, including some that appear to be protective against cancer. Most notable among them is resveratrol, which is discussed on page 186. Hard liquor, on the other hand, adds no nutritive value to your diet. So why bother!

Research also shows that wine drinkers, in general, live healthier lifestyles and tend to drink as part of a meal—a fact that researchers speculate may be the real key to their better health.

Some at-risk people should avoid drinking altogether. This includes women at risk for breast cancer, especially overweight or obese women past menopause, smokers, and people with liver damage, diabetes, and high blood pressure.

DO YOUR PART TO CUT DOWN ON AIR POLLUTION

If you live in or near a city with air pollution, there isn't a whole lot you can do about it, except move. In many ways, air pollution is a part of our existence. Although a lot has been done to reduce emissions levels and pollutants in the air we breathe, air pollution and smog are still major problems in many locales in the United States. On any given day, an estimated 345 monitored counties violate the eight-hour ozone standard of 0.075 parts per million established by the U.S. Environmental Protection Agency (EPA). The poorer the quality of air, the greater your risk of respiratory illness. Studies indicate that pollution is also associated with an increased risk of cancer.

For the sake of your personal health, you should be aware of the quality of the air that you breathe in the places where you live, work and recreate. The EPA has established an Air Quality Index to alert you to the level of harmful pollution in your area or area nearest you. Find out about the quality of your air space by visiting www.epa.gov.

Cities with the highest air pollution levels include:

- Los Angeles
- Bakersfield, CA
- Visalia, CA
- Fresno, CA
- Houston, TX
- Sacramento, CA
- Dallas–Fort Worth, TX

- Charlotte, NC
- Phoenix, AZ
- El Centro, CA

Cities with the cleanest air are:

- Billings, MO
- Carson City, NV
- Coeur d'Alene, ID
- Fargo, SD
- Honolulu, HI
- Laredo, TX
- Lincoln, NE
- Port St. Lucie, FL
- Sioux Falls, SD

The EPA rates air quality and warnings on six color-coded levels, ranging from 50 to 500, which are often publicly posted. Turn the page to determine what they mean.

Emissions Control
Across the board, the biggest contributor to poor air quality is emissions from cars and trucks. You can do your part to reduce this problem by using your automobile less frequently. Here are a few ideas:

- Carpool to work and events involving children's activities.
- Combine all your errands and do them in one or two trips a week.
- Walk instead of drive whenever possible.
- Get a bicycle and use it as an alternative mode of transportation.

- If you're stalled in heavy traffic, turn off your car's engine. Do the same at traffic lights, if traffic allows.
- Consider a hybrid vehicle next time you make an automobile purchase.

CHECK YOUR HOME FOR RADON

The EPA considers radon a national health problem. And for good reason. The Nuclear Regulatory Commission says that a family whose home emits more radon than the acceptable level of 4 pCi/l (meaning picoCuries per liter) is exposed to approximately 35 times as much radiation as they'd be exposed to if they were living next to a radioactive waste site.

So, do you know if living in your house is like living next to a nuclear waste dump? If you don't, then you should do a radon check.

Radon is the second leading cause of lung cancer, next to smoking. This gas, which seeps into homes through the soil, has been found in every type of house in every state in the country. The EPA estimates that 8 million homes in the United States have levels beyond what is considered safe. Radon is odorless and invisible and there are no symptoms to alert you to its presence, so the only way to know the level of radon in your home is to have it tested.

Granite is a secondary source of radon in the home, so if you have granite countertops, mantels or floors, you will need more than one radon kit. Granite contains uranium, a primary source for radon. The EPA says only about 10 percent of granite in homes contains radon, but you should still test for it.

Testing is easy. You can buy a radon testing kit at most hardware stores for $20 or less. All you have to do

AIR QUALITY INDEX

Code	Color	Risk	Warning
50	Green	None	None
51–100	Yellow	Moderate	Highly sensitive people should limit exertion outdoors.
101–150	Orange	Unhealthy for sensitive people	Active children and adults with respiratory illnesses should limit outdoor activities.
151–200	Red	Unhealthy	Active children and adults with respiratory illnesses should avoid outdoor activity; everyone else should limit exertion outdoors.
201–300	Purple	Very unhealthy	Everyone can experience some effects. Those with respiratory problems should avoid the outdoors.
301–500	Maroon	Hazardous	A health warning of emergency proportions that affects all people.

is put it in your basement and leave it for two days. If you have granite in your kitchen or bathroom, place a kit in those rooms, too. If the test shows that radon in your home is above 4pCi/l, you'll need to take action.

Most radon problems can be fixed by installing a ventilating system that will direct the radon away from your house. You most likely will need to hire a contractor who is an expert in radon removal to do this for you. This could cost around $1,500. However, if you're a do-it-yourselfer, you can probably do it for half as much, or less. If you'd prefer the assistance of an expert, look online for a list of "certified radon mitigators" in your state.

If it turns out that your granite countertops are a problem, you'll have to revamp your kitchen or bathroom ventilating system or replace the granite.

GET PROACTIVE ABOUT YOUR HEALTH

All-time-high medical costs have created a new paradigm in the American health care system. Insurance regulations may limit the doctor you want to see. When you go to the doctor, you may not even see your doctor but, rather, a nurse practitioner. When you do get to see a doctor, your visit may be on a time clock.

It all means that it is more important now than ever to take responsibility for your own health care. You no longer can depend on your doctor to send you reminders that your physical is due, or that it's time to get a mammogram or colonoscopy. *You* must be your own best medical watchdog.

It is in your best interest to have a primary care physician who knows as much about your health as you do. He or she should be aware of your family medical history, cancer in your family, and your diet, exercise and lifestyle habits. Discuss risk factors with your doctor and the best time for you to start screening for certain cancers. Know when a routine cancer screening is due and take responsibility for getting the appointment. Most importantly, make sure to call to get the results of screenings and other tests if the office doesn't call you within an appropriate amount of time. Do not assume no news is good news.

Also, don't accept "everything's fine" or "normal." If it's your blood count, ask what the number is and write it down. Never be timid about asking the doctor's office to give you the details you need for your own self-care.

QUESTION YOUR NEED FOR X-RAYS

The National Council on Radiation Protection and Measurement (NCRP) believes many Americans are being overexposed to radiation as a result of medical imaging tests, and in 2007 it inaugurated the "Image Gently" campaign to alert both doctors and patients to weigh the merits of a radiation-exposed procedure before proceeding with it. Your part, as a patient, is to keep a record of your medical X-ray and imaging history and question any doctor ordering a test that exposes you to radiation. This is the NCRP's list of questions and the responses you should be looking for:

- Why do I need this exam?
   For every test, the information learned should lead to an expected benefit, such as a diagnosis or treatment decision.
- How will having this exam improve my health care?
   Having the test should have an impact on the management of your illness.

- Are there alternatives that do not use radiation that are equally as good?

  If there is another test that can produce the same results, you should know about it and get the appropriate background to make an informed choice.

- Do you have any financial interest in the facility where you want me to get this procedure?

  If the answer is anything but no, you should ask even more questions.

  And, if the test is for a child:

- Will my child receive a "kid-sized" radiation dose?

  Children should never to exposed to radiation that is not essential and at levels that are unnecessary. You should also keep a log of all your children's medical tests. You can start one by downloading "My Child's Medical Imaging Record" at www.imagegently.org.

These questions are important because Americans are now being exposed to more than seven times as much ionizing radiation from medical procedures than in the early 1980s. Most of this is from the overuse of CT scans being performed on people who have no symptoms and are at low risk for disease. This is happening for three reasons, according to the NCRP:

Patients making self referrals. This means responding to a third-party advertisement or invitation to get normally uninsured screenings at a reduced rate, as part of a special program. The NCRP recommends that you do this only with the consent of your primary care physician. You should also be assured that the firm and individual performing the test are qualified radiologists.

Fear of litigation. Doctors may feel the need to order a test "just in case," no matter how remote the chances are that something will be found. This could occur in order to establish a paper trail should your case result in a malpractice suit.

Doctors may get a financial kickback. A doctor may be financially invested in a radiology practice to which he or she refers patients. This, says the NCRP, could motivate a doctor to make a referral for a test that is not essential to your diagnosis or treatment options.

Unfortunately, where exposure changes to at-risk overexposure is a gray area, which is why your doctor should be apprised of all referred and self-referred procedures that you get. The HPS recommends that radiation only be used on people at high risk for disease and for whom the test will dictate a diagnosis and/or form of treatment.

SOURCES

This is a selected list from the more than 300 sources used to write this book.

CHAPTER 1

Aggarwal BB, Danda D et al. 2009. Model for prevention and treatment of cancer: Problem vs promises. *Biochemical Pharmacology.* May; 27(9): 2097–116.

Anand Tp. Kunnumakkara AB, et al. 2008. Cancer is a preventable disease that requires major lifestyle changes. *Pharmacology Research.* Sept; 25(9): 2200.

Boyle P, Levin B. 2008. *World Cancer Report 2008.* World Health Organization. Lyon, France.

CHAPTER 2

Boyle P, Levin B. 2008. *World Cancer Report 2008.* World Health Organization. Lyon, France.

Doll R, et al. 1994. Mortality in relation to consumption of alcohol: 13 years' observations on male British doctors. *British Medical Journal.* Oct 8; 309(6959): 911–8.

Doll R, Peto R. 1981. The causes of cancer; quantitative estimates of avoidable risks in the United States today. *Journal of the National Cancer Institute.* 66: 1191–1308.

Franco EL, Harper DM. 2005. Vaccine against human papillomavirus: a new paradigm in cervical cancer control. *Vaccine.* 23: 2388–2394.

Grossman E, et al. 2002. Is there an association between hypertension and cancer mortality? *The American Journal of Medicine.* Apr 15: 112(6): 479–86.

IARC. 2004. *Monographs on the evaluation of carcinogenic risks to humans.* Vol 83. Lyon, France.

Kitto ME, Haines DK, Arauzo HD. 2009. Emanation of radon from household granite. *Health Physics.* Apr; 96(4): 477–82.

Negri E, et al. 2002. Family history of cancer and risk of ovarian cancer. *European Journal of Cancer.* Mar; 39(4): 505–10.

Pandeyta N, Williams G et al. 2009. Alcohol consumption and the risks of adenocarcinoma and squamous cell carcinoma of the esophagus. *Gastroenterology.* Apr; 136(4): 1215–24, e1-2.

Reeves GK, et al. 2007. Cancer incidence and mortality in relation to body mass index in the Million Women Study: cohort study. Dec. 1; 335(7630): 1134.

Siegel M and Skeer M. 2003. Exposure to secondhand smoke and excess lung cancer mortality risk among workers in the "5 Bs": bars, bowling alleys, billiard halls, betting establishments and bingo parlors. *Tobacco Control.* 12: 333–338.

Siegel M, Barbeau EM, Osinubi OY. 2006. The impact of tobacco use and secondhand smoke on hospitality workers. *Clinics in Occupational and Environmental Medicine.* 5(1): 31–42.

CHAPTER 3

Mandelson MT et al. 2000. Breast density as a predictor of mammographic detection: comparison of interval- and screen-detected cancers. *Jounral of the National Cancer Institute.* Jul 5; 92(13): 1081–7.

Mayo Clinic office visit. 2009. Molecular breast imaging. *Mayo Clinic Women's HealthSource.* Mar.; 13(3): 6.

Piturro M. 2008. Diagnosing and treating oral cancer. *The Wall Street Journal.* Mar 7–8: A6C.

CHAPTER 4

Bosetti C et al. 2002. Olive oil, seed oils and other added fats in relation to ovarian cancer (Italy). *Cancer Causes Control.* Jun: 13(5): 465–70.

De Moreno, de LeBlanc. 2007. The application of probiotics in cancer. *British Journal of Nutrition.* Oct; 98 Suppl 1: S105–10.

Ding H et al. 2007. Chemopreventive characteristics of avocado fruit. *Seminars in Cancer Biology.* Oct; 17(5): 286–94.

Fang N, et al. 2006. Inhibition of growth and induction of apoptosis in human cancer cell lines by an ethyl acetate fraction from shiitake mushrooms. *Journal of Alternative Complementary Medicine.* Mar; 12(2): 124–32.

Galeone C, Pelucchi C et al. 2009. Allium vegetables intake and endometrial cancer risk. *Public Health and Nutrition.* Sept; 12(9): 1576–9.

Galeone C, Pelucchi C et al. 2006. Onion and garlic use and human cancer. *The American Journal of Clinical Nutrition.* Nov; 84(5): 1027–32.

Hangen L, Bennick MR. 2002. Consumption of black beans and navy beans (Phaseolus vulgaris) reduced azoxymethane-induced colon cancer in rats. *Nutrition and Cancer.* 44(1):60–5.

Hardman WE. 2007. Dietary canola oil suppressed growth of implanted MDA-MB 231 human breast tumors in nude mice. *Nutrition and Cancer.* 57(2): 177–83.

Hong MY, Seeram NP, Heber D. 2008. Pomegranate polyphenols down-regulate expression of androgen-synthesizing genes in human prostate cancer cells overexpressing the androgen receptor. *Journal of Nutritional Biochemistry.* Dec;19(12):848–55.

Horn-Ross OL et al. 2003. Phytoestrogen intake and endometrial cancer risk. *Journal of the National Cancer Institute.* Aug 6;95(15):1158–64.

Jedrychowski W, Maugeri U. 2008. Protective effect of fish consumption on colorectal cancer risk. Hospital-based case-control study in Eastern Europe. *Annals of Nutritional Metabolism.* 53(3-4): 295–302. Epub 2009 Jan 26.

Jin YR, Less MS et al. 2007. Intake of vitamin A-rich foods and lung cancer risk in Taiwan: with special reference to garland chrysanthemum and sweet potato leaf consumption. *Asian Pacific Journal of Clinical Nutrition.* 16(3): 377–88.

Larsson SC, Andersson So., Johansson JE, Wolk A et al. 2008. Cultured milk, yogurt, and dairy intake in relation to bladder cancer risk in a prospective study of Swedish women and men. Oct; 88(4):1083–87.

Lee SA, Shu XO et al. 2009. Adolescent and adult soy food intake and breast cancer risk: results from the Shanghai Women's Health Study. *American Journal of Clinical Nutrition.* April. Epub ahead of print.

Liu J, Xing J, Fei Y. 2008. Green tea (Camellia sinensis) and cancer prevention: a systematic review of randomized trials and epidemiological studies. *Chinese Medicine.* Oct 22; 3:12.

Ng ML, Yap, et al. 2002. Inhibition of human colon carcinoma development by lentinan from shiitake mushrooms (Lentinus edodes). *Journal of Alternative Complementary Medicine.* Oct; 8(5): 581–9.

Ngo SN, William DB, Cobiac L, Head RJ. 2007. Does garlic reduce risk of colorectal cancer? A systematic review. *The Journal of Nutrition.* Oct;137(10): 2264–9.

Owen RW, Haubner R et al. 2004. Olives and olive oil in cancer prevention. *European Journal of Cancer Prevention.* Aug;13(4): 219–26.

Prasad S, Kalra N, Shukla Y. 2008. Induction of apoptosis by lupeol and mango extract in mouse prostate and LNCaP cells. *Nutrition and Cancer.* 60(1):120–30.

Sofi F et al. 2008. Adherence to Mediterranean diet and health status: meta-analysis. *British Medical Journal.* Sept. 11; 337.

Stoner GD, Wang LS, Casto BC. 2008. Laboratory and clinical studies of cancer chemoprevention by antioxidants in berries. *Carcinogenesis.* Sept;29(9):1665–74.

Verhagen H et al. 1995. Reduction of oxidative DNA damage in humans by Brussels sprouts. *Carcinogenesis.* Apr;16(4): 969–70.

Zhang J, Nagasaki M, et al. 2003. Capsaicin inhibits growth of adult T-cell leukemia cells. *Leukemia Research.* Mar; 27(3): 275–83.

CHAPTER 5

Athar M, Back JH et al. 2007. Resveratrol: a review of preclinical studies for human cancer prevention. *Toxicology and Applied Pharmacology.* Nov 1; 224(3): 274–83.

Chen J, Stavro PM, Thompson LU. 2002. Dietary flaxseed inhibits human breast cancer growth and metastasis and downregulates expression of insulin-like growth factor and epidermal growth factor receptor. *Nutrition and Cancer.* 43:187–92.

Chen Q, Espey MG et al. 2005. Pharmacologic ascorbic acid concentrations selectively kill cancer cells: action as a pro-drug to deliver hydrogen peroxide to tissues. *Proceeding of the National Academy of Sciences of the United States.* Sep 20;102(38):13604–9.

E-Serag HB, Lagergren J. 2009. Alcohol drinking and the risk of Barrett's esophagus and esophageal adenocarcinoma. *Gastroenterology.* April;136(4):1155–7.

Eynard AR, Lopez CB. 2003. Conjugated linoleic acid (CLA) versus saturated fats/cholesterol: their proportion in fatty and lean meats may affect the risk of developing colon cancer. *Lipids in Health and Disease.* Aug 29; 2:6.

Flossmann E, Rothwell PM. 2007. Effect of aspirin on long-term risk of colorectal cancer: consistent evidence from randomized and observational studies. *Lancet.* 369:1603–1613.

Gali-Muhtasib H., Diab-Assaf M, Boltze C, Al-Hmaira J. 2004. Thymoquinone extracted from black seed triggers apoptotic cell death in human colorectal cancer cells via a p53-dependent mechanism. *International Journal of Oncology.* Oct; 25(4): 857–66.

Ip C, Lisk DJ, Stoewsand GS. 1992. Mammary cancer prevention by regular garlic and selenium-enriched garlic. *Nutrition and Cancer.* 17(3): 279–86.

Ip MM, Masso-Welch PA, Ip C. 2003. Prevention of mammary cancer with conjugated linoleic acid: role of the stroma and the epithelium. *Journal of Mammary Gland Biology and Neoplasia.* Jan; 8(1):103–108.

Karppi J, Kurl S et al. 2009. Serum Lycopene and the Risk of Cancer: The Kuopio Ischaemic Heart Disease Risk Factor (KIHD) Study. *Annals of Epidemiology.* May 12 e-pub.

Lee KW, Lww HJ, Surh YJ, Lee CY. 2003. Vitamin C and cancer chemoprevention: reappraisal. *The American Journal of Clinical Nutrition.* Dec; 8(6):1074–8.

Lin X, Gingrich JR, Bao W, Li J, Haroon ZA, Demark-Wahnefried W. 2002. Effect of flaxseed supplementation on prostatic carcinoma in transgenic mice. *Urology.* 60: 919–24.

Shin HR, Kim JY et al. 2000. The cancer-preventive potential of Panax ginseng: a review of human and experimental evidence. *Cancer Causes and Control.* Jul;11(6): 55–76.

Slattery ML, Benson J et al. 2000. Carotenoids and colon cancer. *American Journal of Clinical Nutrition.* Feb; 71(2): 575–82.

Surbsole MJ, Jim F et al. 2001. Dietary folate intake and breast cancer risk: results from the Shanghai Breast Cancer Study. *Cancer Research.* Ocr 1;61(19):7136–41.

Thomson M, Ali M. 2003. Garlic [Allium sativum]: a review of its potential use as an anti-cancer agent. *Current Cancer Drug Targets.* Feb; 3(1): 67–81.

Wang, Y, et al. 2006. The red wine polyphenol resveratrol displays bilevel inhibition on aromatase in breast cancer cells. *Toxicology Science.* July; 92(1):71–7.

CHAPTER 6
Kitto ME, Haines DK, Arauzo HD. 2009. Emanation of radon from household granite. *Health Physics.* Apr; 96(4): 477–82.